Infused Waters

Infused Waters

50 SIMPLE DRINKS TO
RESTORE, REVIVE & RELAX

GEORGINA DAVIES

Photography by Luke Albert

Hardie Grant

QUADRILLE

CONTENTS

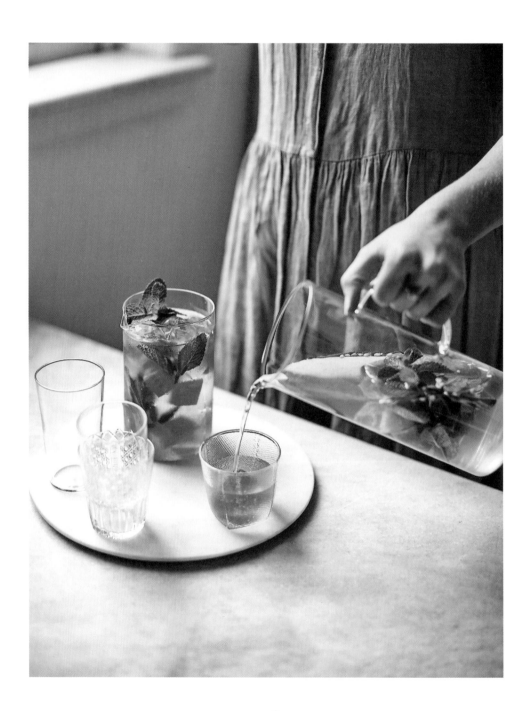

INTRODUCTION

We all know we should be drinking more water. At least two litres a day, the experts recommend. But how many of us can say, hand on hearts, that we have no trouble downing that every 24 hours?

Instead we're more likely to find ourselves lured by flavourful beverages containing alcohol, caffeine, sugars or sweeteners which, while making our tastebuds zing, can also make the rest of our bodies lag.

As anyone trying to beat the booze, curb the coffee or ditch the diet cola will know, boring, plain old water hardly makes a satisfying substitute for such tastier concoctions.

Or does it? This book aims to demonstrate that H_2O can be so much more. Adding fruits, herbs, vegetables and spices to a simple glass of cold or hot water does wonders to improve the taste, opening up a whole new world of flavours.

But that's not all. It also introduces a host of health benefits, from helping with digestion and metabolism and therefore aiding healthy weight management, to providing vital vitamins to nurture the immune system.

Hydration is key for maintaining every system in our body. It improves skin and hair health, keeping complexions clear and nourished, while also boosting brain power, preventing headaches and making it easier to think clearly.

The restorative, reviving and relaxing recipes you'll find in these pages aim to make staying well-hydrated simple and tasty. Quick and easy, and using an exciting range of herbs, fruits, vegetables and spices, they add a flavourful, healthy and original spark to the humble glass of water.

A FEW TIPS TO GET YOU STARTED

INGREDIENTS

- When possible, buy good quality produce.

- Ensure all fruit, vegetables and herbs are washed before use.

- Use unwaxed citrus fruit. (Unwaxed lemons are widely available from supermarkets. Unfortunately, you can probably assume that all other citrus fruits *do* have a wax coating. To easily remove the wax, place the fruit in a colander set over the sink and carefully pour over very hot water. Gently scrub the peel with a stiff brush then rinse the fruit in cold water and dry.)

- Use fresh herbs, unless otherwise stated.

- All fruit and vegetables should be left unpeeled, unless otherwise stated.

- Leave fruit such as apples and pears uncored, unless otherwise stated.

- Always grind spices from fresh, unless otherwise stated.

- Use filtered water when possible.

- Feel free to experiment: try using sparkling water instead of still. Or serve cold infusions over ice.

QUANTITIES

- All water quantities are measured in US cups. For a metric conversion use one US cup = 250ml.

- All cold infusion recipes make five cups or a 1.25-litre jugful. All hot infusion recipes make two cups or 500ml – enough to fill a small teapot.

- In all cases this should be sufficient to serve two to three people, unless otherwise stated.

- To make a generous portion for one person, or enough to fill a regular-sized water bottle, halve the ingredients of the cold infusions.

- The instructions given explain how to create infusions in a large vessel, but feel free to make them in individual glasses or mugs, if you like.

- Most cold recipes need to infuse for at least two hours. If making in a water bottle to take to work or the gym, make your chosen drink the night before and leave to infuse overnight. You can, of course, serve infusions straight away if you like, but the flavours will be less intense.

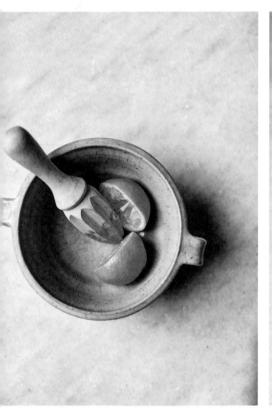
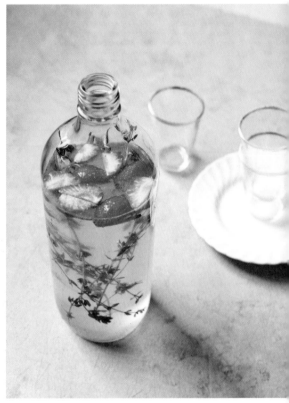

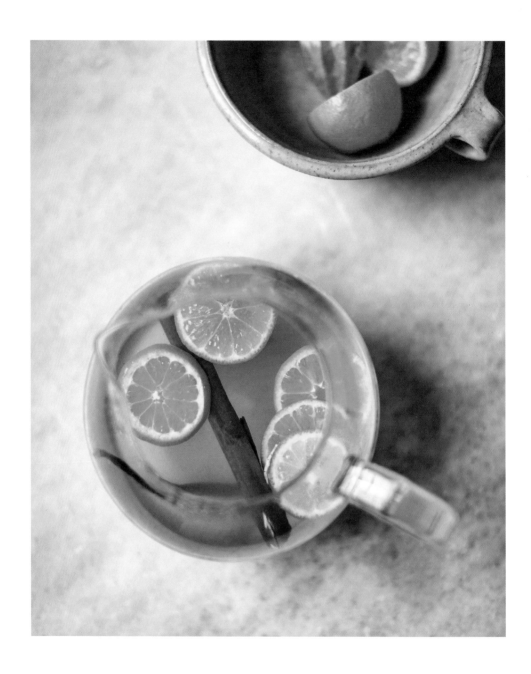

INGREDIENT HEALTH BENEFITS

FRUITS

Apples are low in fruit sugars but high in vitamins, making them perfect to use in infused waters. They're full of antioxidants and dietary fibre and are great at speeding up the metabolism.

Beetroot (beet) helps to detoxify the liver. It has a diverse nutritional profile, rich in calcium, iron and vitamins A and C.

Blueberries may be small but pack a serious punch healthwise – they are bursting with nutrients, antioxidants and vitamin C which help to protect your cells and look after your heart.

Cucumber contains skin-boosting nutrients. They're also great at treating darkness and puffiness around the eyes.

Fennel aids bone health, blood pressure regulation and heart health. It's also great for reducing water retention and regulating your digestion.

Kiwis contain the enzyme actinidain, which aids digestion. They're also packed with immune-boosting vitamins.

Lemon is a great source of vitamin C, aids digestion and freshens breath. A simple slice in a mug of hot water is the perfect way to start your day and gently wake up your digestive system.

Oranges are one of nature's richest sources of vitamin C, a powerful antioxidant that helps to protect our cells. Use them in your infused waters to help ward off colds and flu.

Pineapple is high in vitamin C and antioxidants, a great immune system support, and helps ward off colds.

Pomegranates are rich in vitamins C, K and B (especially folate) and pack a big antioxidant punch. B vitamins are important in repairing DNA, while other health benefits of pomegranates also include reduced inflammation in the gut and improved digestion.

Strawberries are an excellent source of vitamins K and C, and provide a good dose of fibre, folic acid and potassium. As with all berries, they're best eaten when in season.

HERBS

Basil is anti-inflammatory and helps promote good liver health. It is also rich in magnesium, which helps blood flow, and has some antibacterial properties.

Camomile is soothing and healing with anti-inflammatory properties that can relieve skin irritations. Its calming effects can also help induce a peaceful night's sleep.

Lemon balm is widely known for its calming properties and helps ease stress and anxiety. Perfect to aid a good night's sleep.

Lemon grass is antibacterial and great for fighting bad breath, as well as warding off infection.

Mint is a soothing herb that aids digestion and helps support healthy cholesterol levels.

Rosehip is rich in vitamin C, so is perfect for preventing colds and viruses. Drinking rosehip tea also helps to nourish the skin, reducing signs of aging.

Rosemary is a fragrant, calming herb and a rich source of iron, calcium and vitamin B.

Thyme is another great herb to aid digestion – its natural oils can also help soothe coughs and sore throats.

SPICES

Cardamom is packed full of antioxidants, helping lower blood pressure, and can also boost digestive health, alleviating indigestion and nausea.

Cinnamon helps lower blood sugar levels and contains many antiviral, antibacterial and antifungal properties.

Ginger can treat any form of nausea and so help ward off morning or travel sickness. It strengthens the digestive system and can alleviate heartburn.

Turmeric has powerful antibacterial, antioxidant and anti-inflammatory properties and has long been used to treat and prevent many ailments. It boosts digestion and helps ward off bugs and viruses.

Star anise helps alleviate nausea, improves digestion and soothes coughs and sore throats.

Vanilla can help reduce unhealthy cholesterol levels and contains essential oils that strengthen hair and nails.

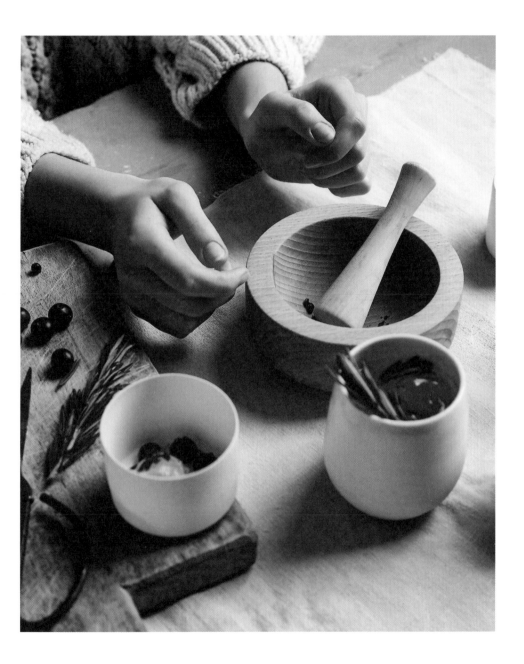

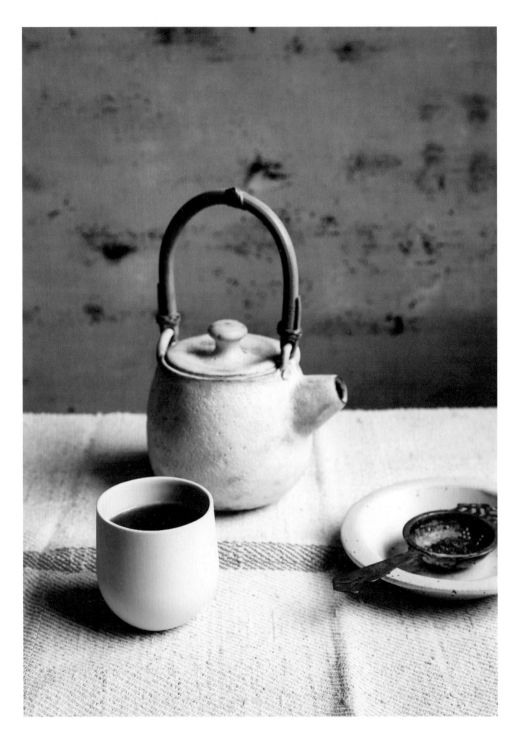

FROM THE PANTRY

Apple cider vinegar is a health-boosting ingredient for many reasons. It helps balance your body's pH levels, aids digestion, helps control blood pressure and enables your body to absorb more nutrients from food. Make sure you buy a brand that still contains 'the mother' – all the beneficial enzymes and good bacteria, or probiotics, of the unfiltered raw vinegar.

Honey is nature's energy booster. Containing antibacterial compounds, it's the perfect natural replacement for your usual sweetener. Cheap supermarket honey is often full of added sugar, so it's worth splashing out on the good stuff. If you suffer from hay fever, using honey that is local to your area can help to reduce symptoms – it's also lovely to support local beekeepers.

Rose water helps sooth digestive ailments, as well as having anti-aging and skin-boosting properties.

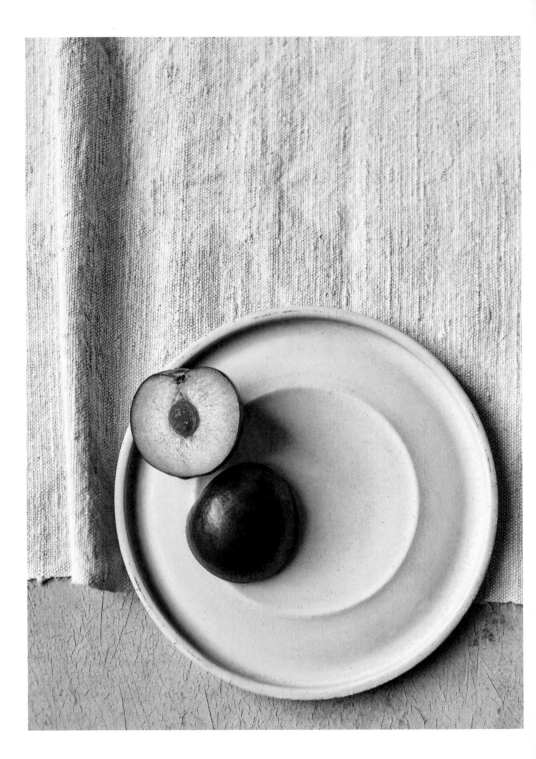

RESTORE

The recipes in this chapter focus on soothing, restorative ingredients. From ginger and apple cider vinegar, both known for their gut-healing properties, to mellow fruits and calming botanicals, these ingredients all add that little something extra to a glass of hot or cold water to give you a boost.

BLACKBERRY, ORANGE & GINGER

INGREDIENTS
10 blackberries
1 orange
1 thumb of ginger
5 cups of water
ice, optional

METHOD
In a small bowl, bruise the blackberries slightly with the back of a spoon, then scrape them into a large jug along with any juice. Finely zest the orange, slice it, then add everything to the jug. Thinly slice the ginger and pop that in, too. Fill the jug with the cold water and leave to infuse in the fridge for at least two hours before drinking. Serve over ice, if you like, for a refreshing infusion.

TIP
When in season, use blood oranges to create an even prettier infusion.

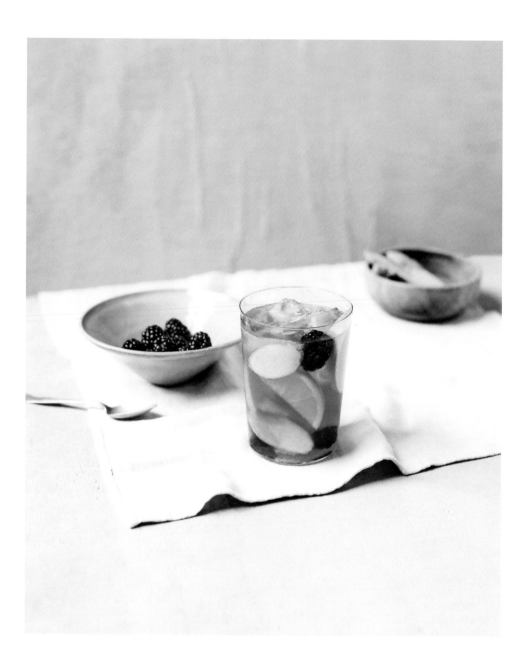

GINGER & MELON

INGREDIENTS
$\frac{1}{2}$ a honeydew melon
2 thumbs of ginger
5 cups of sparkling water

METHOD
Remove the skin from the melon, chop the flesh into large chunks then pop into a large jug. Thinly slice the ginger, add this to the melon and then fill the jug up with sparkling water. Leave to infuse in the fridge for at least two hours before drinking.

TIP
To keep ginger fresh, store it in the freezer in slices or thumb-sized chunks. You can use it straight from frozen.

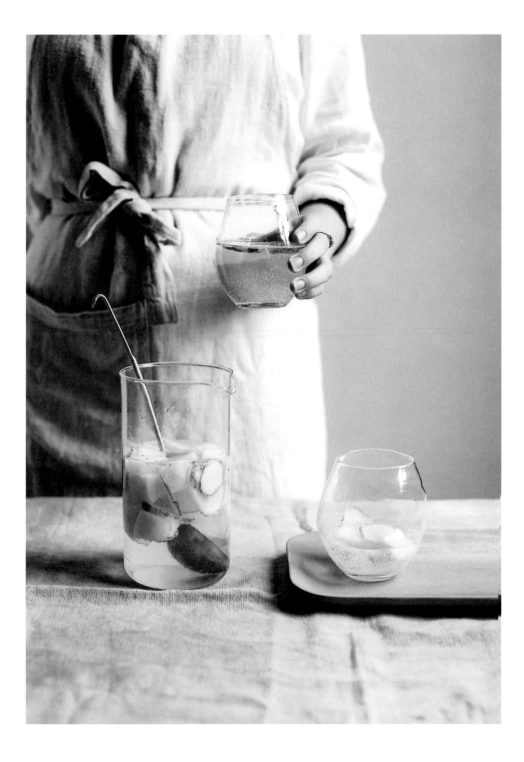

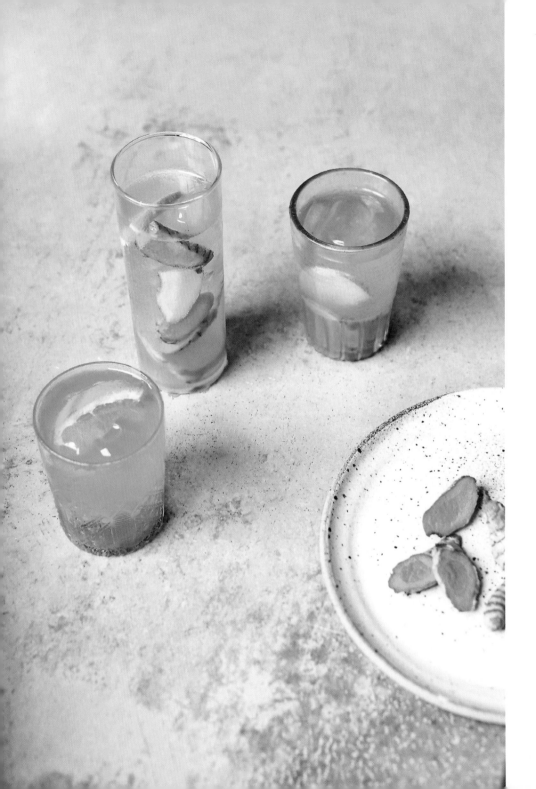

TURMERIC, GINGER & ORANGE

INGREDIENTS
1 thumb of ginger
3 thumbs of fresh
    turmeric
1 orange
5 cups of water
ice, optional

METHOD
Finely slice the ginger and turmeric and scatter them into a large jug. Thinly slice the orange and add this to the jug too. Fill the jug with the cold water and leave to infuse in the fridge for at least two hours before drinking. Super-zingy, especially if served over ice, this is a perfect way to start the day.

TIP
Fresh turmeric is now available from some supermarkets, so it shouldn't be too difficult to get hold of. If your local store doesn't stock it, try a health food store or Asian supermarket.

If you can't get hold of fresh turmeric, substitute it with 1 tsp of ground turmeric; mix it with a little water to form a paste before combining it with the rest of the water.

Be careful when using both fresh and ground turmeric as it stains hands, clothes and work tops easily!

APPLE CIDER VINEGAR & CINNAMON

HOT

INGREDIENTS

2 cinnamon sticks,
    plus extra for serving
    if desired
1 tbsp apple cider vinegar
2 cups of boiling water

METHOD

Lightly crush the cinnamon sticks in a pestle and mortar so they start to release their fragrance. Put the cinnamon and apple cider vinegar in a small teapot and fill with the boiling water. Leave to infuse for five to ten minutes before serving. Breathe in the sweet-smelling steam for ultimate restoration.

TIP

Buy apple cider vinegar that still contains 'the mother' – the beneficial unfiltered enzymes and probiotics. This is a great drink for soothing digestion after a heavy meal.

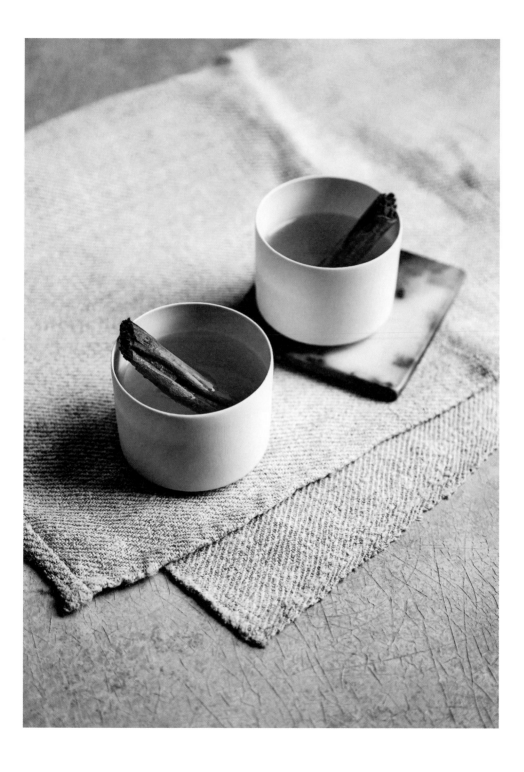

BLUEBERRY, ROSEMARY & JUNIPER

INGREDIENTS
4 juniper berries
15 blueberries
4 sprigs of rosemary,
   plus extra for serving
   if desried
5 cups of water
ice, optional

METHOD
In a pestle and mortar, crush the juniper berries to release their fragrance. Add the blueberries and crush them slightly, too. Pop the mixture into a large jug, then add the rosemary and fill up with the cold water. Leave to infuse in the fridge for at least two hours, then serve with some blueberries a sprig of rosemary in each glass, if you like.

TIP
Juniper berries are commonly used to flavour gin, but are also an ideal ingredient for infusions when you're fighting off an illness as they contain many antiseptic properties.

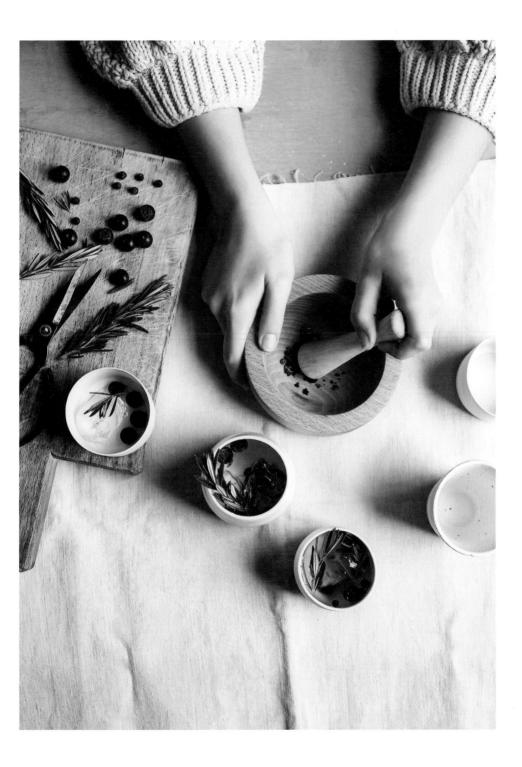

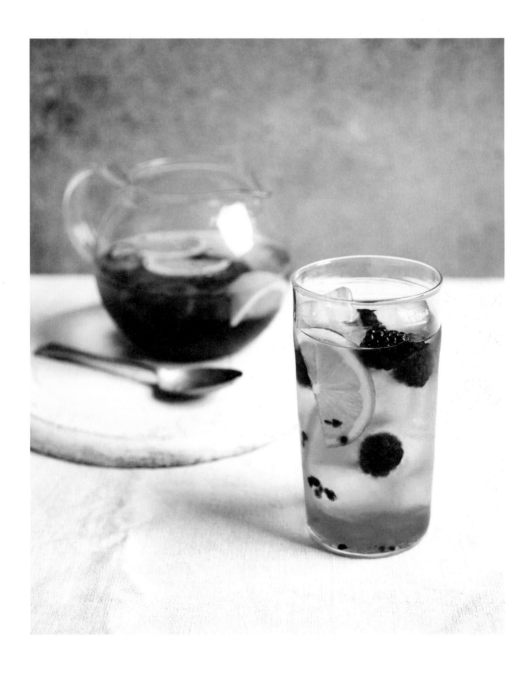

BLACKBERRY & LEMON

INGREDIENTS
10 blackberries
2 lemons
5 cups of water
ice, optional

METHOD
In a small bowl, lightly crush the blackberries with
the back of a spoon then transfer them to a large jug,
making sure to scrape in all the juice. Thinly slice one
of the lemons and add it to the jug with the blackberries.
Squeeze the juice of the remaining lemon into the jug
then add the cold water. Leave to infuse in the fridge for
at least two hours before drinking.

TIP
*For a zingier drink, zest the
lemon before slicing and add
that to your jug, too.*

WATERMELON & MINT

INGREDIENTS
150g (1 cup) rindless,
    chopped watermelon
6 sprigs of mint
5 cups of water
ice, optional

METHOD
Place the chopped watermelon flesh in a large jug.
Lightly crush the sprigs of mint in your hands to release
their fragrance, then add them to the melon. Fill the
jug with the cold water then leave to infuse in the fridge
for at least two hours before drinking. The perfect
thirst-quencher for a hot summer day.

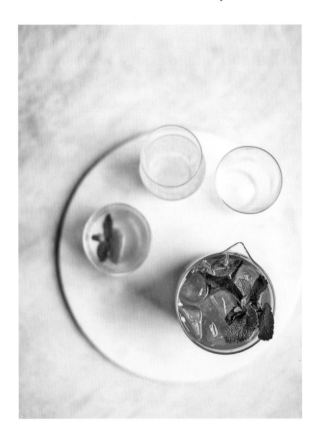

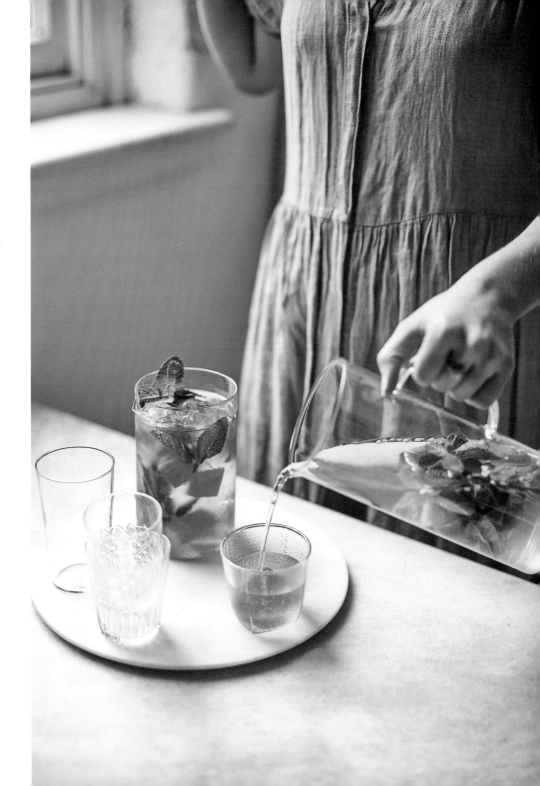

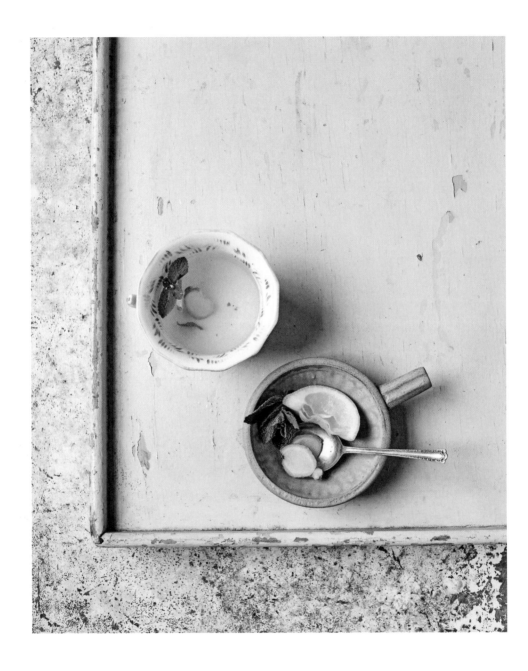

MINT, LEMON & GINGER

HOT

INGREDIENTS
1 thumb of ginger
1 lemon
5 sprigs of mint, plus
   extra for serving
   if desired
2 cups of boiling water

METHOD
Thinly slice the ginger, bruise it slightly using a pestle and mortar then place in a small teapot. Thinly slice the lemon then add to the teapot. Lightly crush the sprigs of mint in your hands to release their fragrance, then add to the other ingredients. Fill the teapot with the boiling water and leave to infuse for five to ten minutes. Serve with a sprig of fresh mint in each cup, if you like.

TIP
Chop up and freeze any leftover fresh herbs. They will lose their vibrant green colour, but are still great for adding flavour to infusions.

STRAWBERRY & THYME

INGREDIENTS
10 strawberries
5 sprigs of thyme,
    plus extra for serving
    if desired
5 cups of water

METHOD
Hull and half the strawberries and pop them in a large jug. Lightly crush the thyme sprigs in your hands to release their fragrance and oils, then place them in the jug alongside the strawberries. Add the cold water and leave to infuse in the fridge for at least two hours. Serve each glass with a fresh sprig of thyme, if you like.

TIP
There are a number of different thyme varieties. For a change, try making this infusion with lemon thyme.

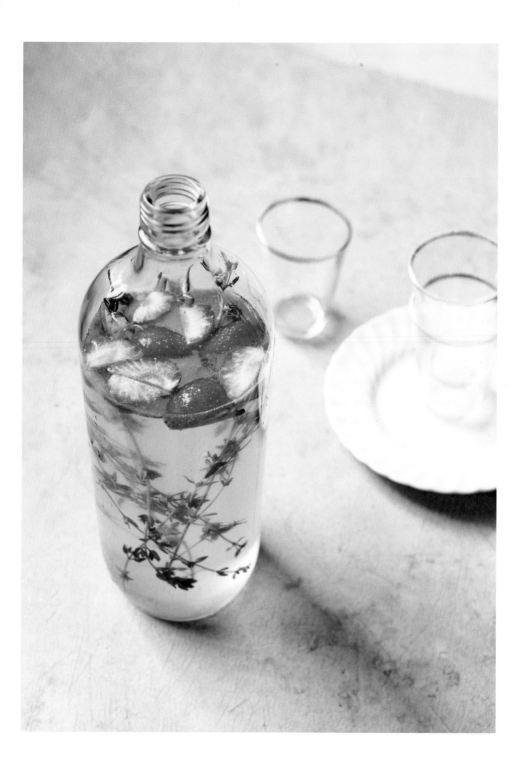

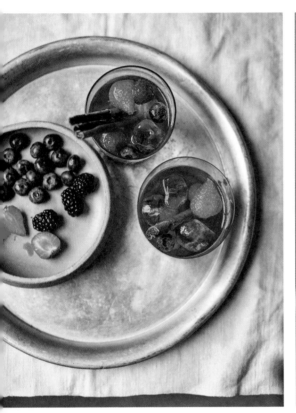
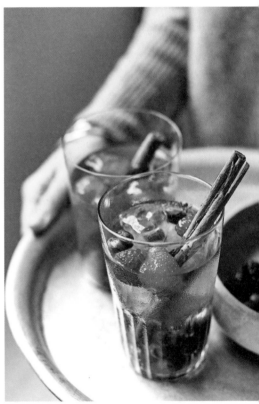

MIXED BERRY & CINNAMON

INGREDIENTS
10 blueberries
10 raspberries
4 strawberries
2 cinnamon sticks,
    plus extra for serving
    if desired
5 cups of water
ice, optional

METHOD
In a small bowl, bruise the blueberries and raspberries lightly with the back of a spoon, then scrape them into a large jug along with any juice. Hull and half the strawberries and add these to the jug. Lightly crush the cinnamon sticks in a pestle and mortar, so that they start to release their fragrance, then pop in the jug along with the berries. Add the cold water and leave to infuse in the fridge for at least two hours. When serving, garnish each glass with a variety of berries and a cinnamon stick, if you like.

TIP
Buy frozen berries when they aren't in season. Most supermarkets do great mixed bags that are really cost-effective, too.

NUTMEG
& GINGER

HOT

INGREDIENTS
2 thumbs of ginger
$\frac{1}{4}$ a whole nutmeg
2 cups of boiling water

METHOD
Thinly slice the ginger, bruise it slightly using a pestle and mortar then place in a small teapot. Grate the nutmeg over the crushed ginger, then fill the teapot with the boiling water and leave to infuse for five to ten minutes before drinking.

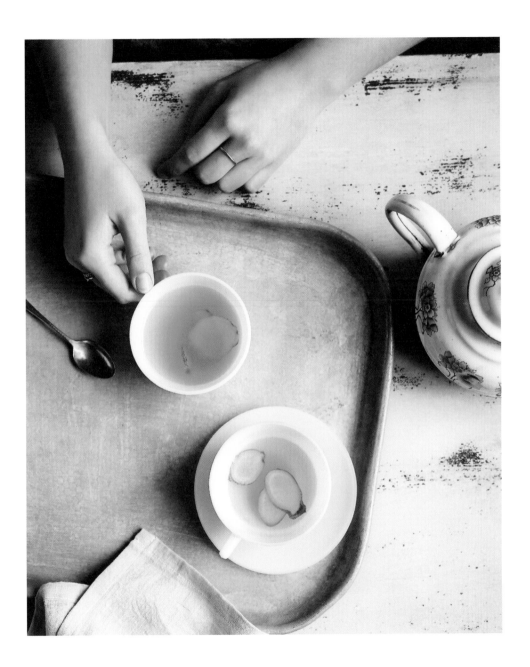

BLACKBERRY, CLEMENTINE & CLOVE

HOT

INGREDIENTS
8 blackberries
4 cloves
2 clementines
2 cups of water

METHOD
In a small bowl, crush the blackberries with the back of a spoon. Scrape the crushed blackberries, along with their juice, into a small saucepan, then add the cloves. Thinly slice one of the clementines and add this to the pan. Cut the remaining clementine in half, squeeze the juice over everything, then add the water. Simmer over a low heat for five to ten minutes then carefully pour into mugs before drinking.

Alternatively, place all of the prepared ingredients in a small teapot, pour over two cups of boiling water and leave to infuse for five to ten minutes.

TIP
This infusion is perfect for the winter months when clementines are in season and at their best. Drink while nibbling on a warm mince pie to restore your sanity after a long day of Christmas shopping.

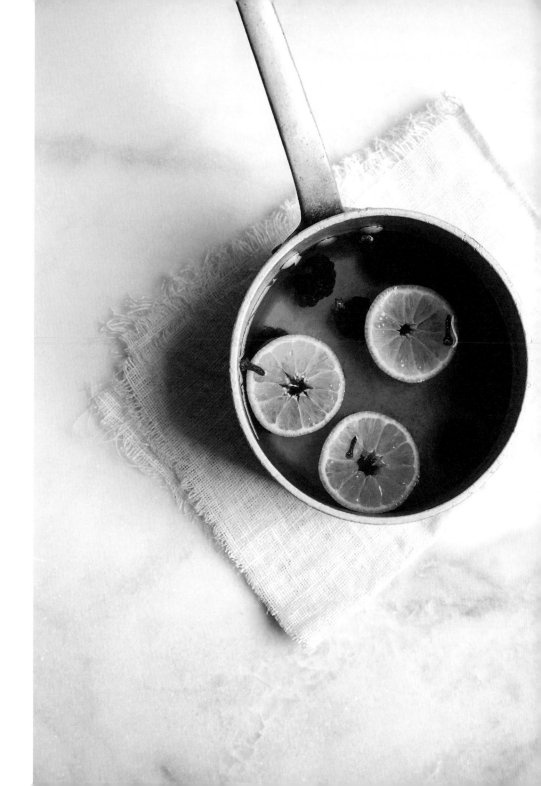

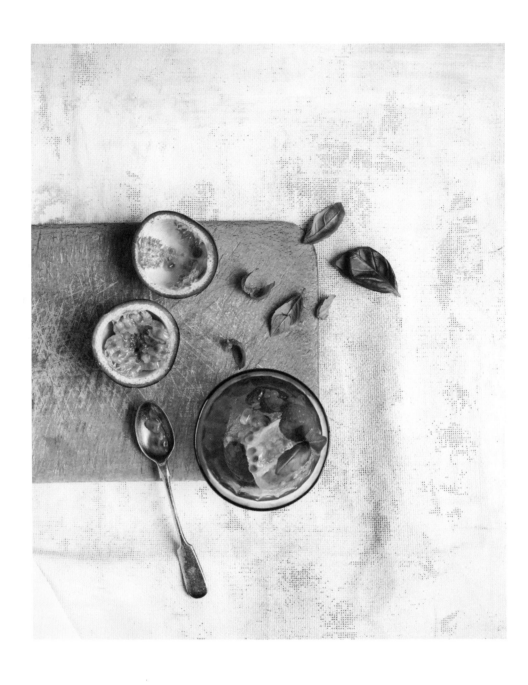

RASPBERRY, PASSION FRUIT & BASIL

INGREDIENTS
15 raspberries
1 passion fruit
5 sprigs of basil,
  plus extra for serving
  if desired
5 cups of water
ice, optional

METHOD
In a small bowl, crush the raspberries gently with the back of a spoon then scrape them into a large jug along with all their juice. Slice the passion fruit in half and scoop the flesh and seeds into the jug. Add the basil, then the cold water. Leave to infuse for at least two hours in the fridge, then serve with a sprig of fresh basil in each glass, if you like.

PLUM & GINGER

HOT

INGREDIENTS
1 thumb of ginger
2 plums
2 cups of water

METHOD
Thinly slice the ginger, bruise it slightly using a pestle and mortar then place in a small saucepan. Slice the plums in half, remove the stones, then thinly slice each half and add to the pan. Add the water to the pan and simmer over a low heat for five to ten minutes before serving.

Alternatively, place the sliced ginger and plums in a small teapot, pour over two cups of boiling water and leave to infuse for five to ten minutes. An ideal restorative for long autumn days.

TIP
Use a mix of different varieties of plums to create a wonderful contrast of colour and sweet and sour flavours.

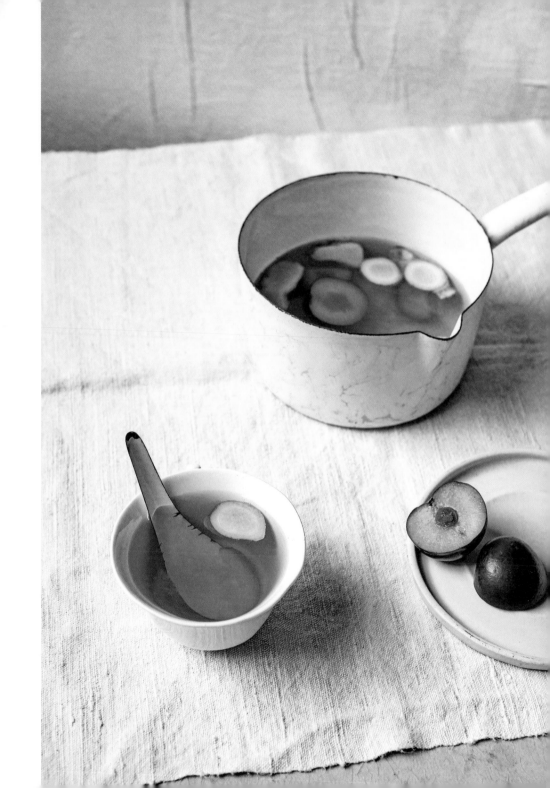

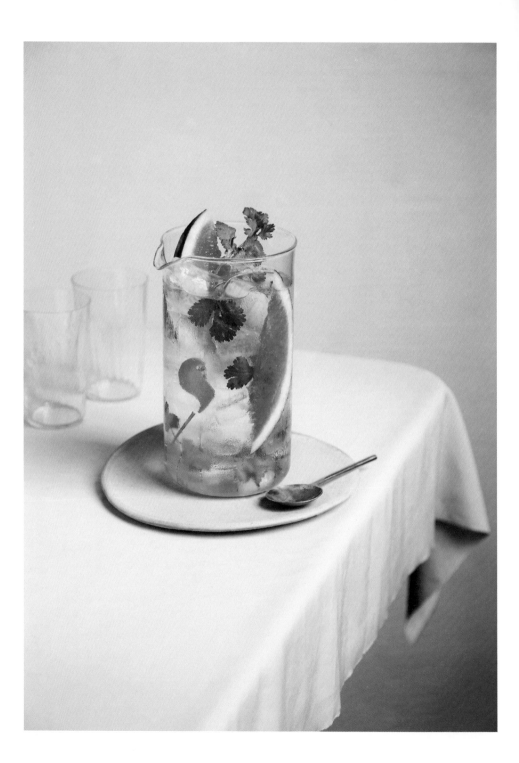

WATERMELON & CORIANDER

INGREDIENTS
½ a small watermelon
10 sprigs of coriander
  (cilantro), plus extra
  for serving if desired
1 orange
5 cups of water
ice, optional

METHOD
Without removing the rind, slice the watermelon half into two large pieces. Place these in a large jug along with the coriander. Thickly zest the orange with a paring knife, add this to the jug, then fill the jug with the cold water. Leave to infuse in the fridge for at least two hours before serving with a sprig of coriander in each glass, if you like.

TIP
To ensure your watermelon is ripe, knock on it with the back of a finger. If it sounds hollow, it's ready to add to your infusion.

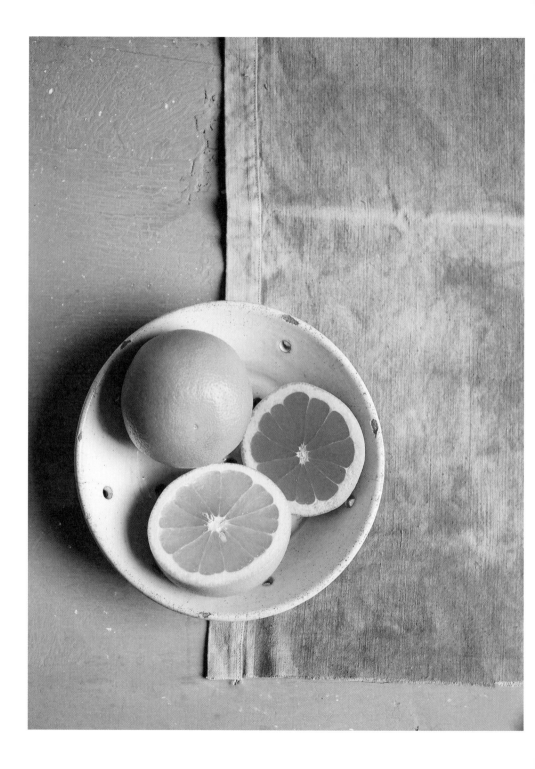

REVIVE

Ensure the perfect start to a busy day with these revitalising recipes. Combining zingy citruses and tropical fruits with perky herbs and botanicals, these uplifting drinks will help you feel your best and think more clearly.

THREE CITRUS

INGREDIENTS
2 oranges
1 pink grapefruit
1 lemon
5 cups of water

METHOD
Squeeze the juice of one of the oranges and half of the grapefruit into a large jug. Thinly slice the other orange, the remaining grapefruit half and the lemon and add these to the jug, too. Add the cold water and leave to infuse in the fridge for at least two hours before drinking.

TIP
Experiment with different citrus fruits – lime will add more of a tang, whereas blood oranges will give your infusion a more dramatic appearance.

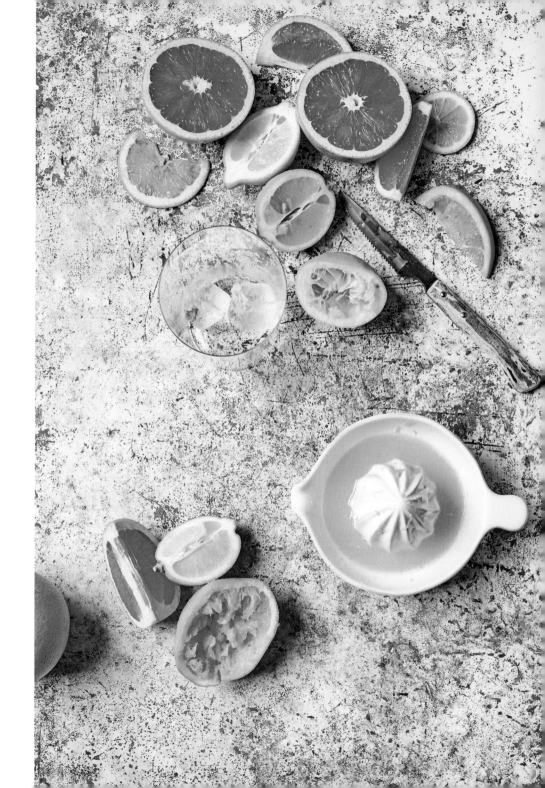

APPLE
& MINT

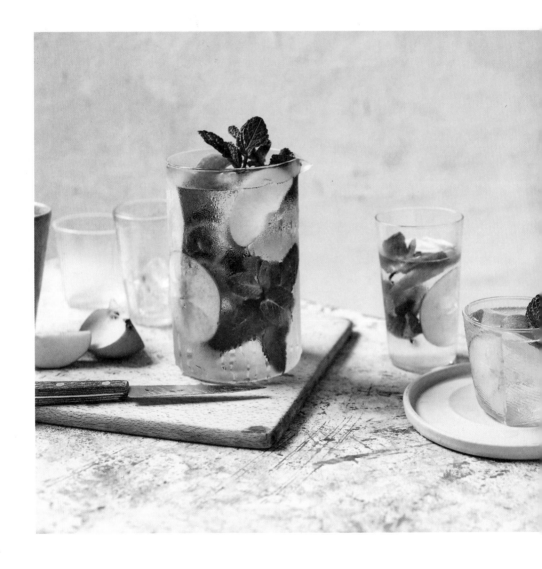

INGREDIENTS
2 apples
10 sprigs of mint, plus extra for serving if desired
5 cups of water
ice, optional

METHOD
Leaving the skin on, slice the apples into wedges and place them in a large jug. Lightly crush the sprigs of mint in your hands to release their fragrance, then add them to the apple. Add the cold water and leave to infuse in the fridge for at least two hours. Serve each glass with a sprig of mint, if you like.

TIP
Crisp apples are best for this infusion. Try Granny Smith for a tart, refreshing drink or Gala if you have more of a sweet tooth.

MANGO &
PASSION FRUIT

HOT

INGREDIENTS
½ a passion fruit
½ a mango
2 cups of boiling water

METHOD
Cut the passion fruit in half and scoop the flesh and seeds of one half into a small teapot. Slice the mango half and add this to the passion fruit seeds. Fill the teapot with the boiling water and leave to infuse for five to ten minutes before drinking.

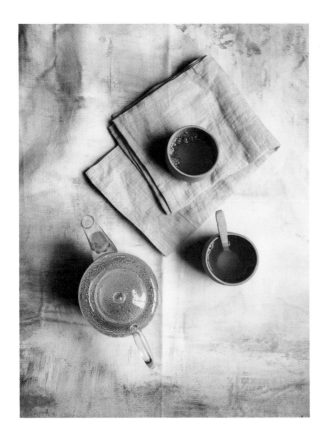

TIP
Peel and slice the remaining mango half and serve it with a squeeze of lime and a sprinkling of chilli salt for the perfect snack to accompany this infusion.

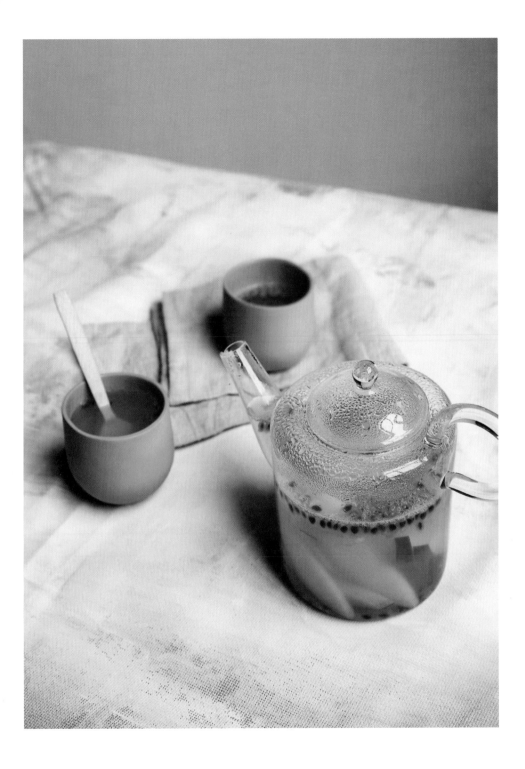

CHERRY & MINT

INGREDIENTS

10 cherries
10 sprigs of mint,
   plus extra for serving
   if desired
5 cups of water
ice, optional

METHOD

Slice the cherries in half, remove their stones, then pop them in a large jug. Lightly crush the sprigs of mint in your hands to release their fragrance, then add them to the cherries. Fill the jug with the cold water, then leave to infuse in the fridge for at least two hours. Serve with a sprig of mint in each glass, if you like.

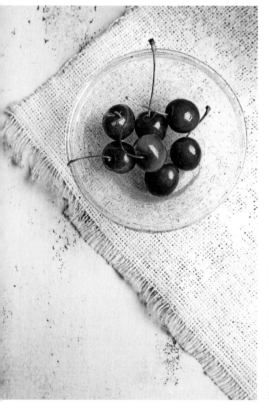

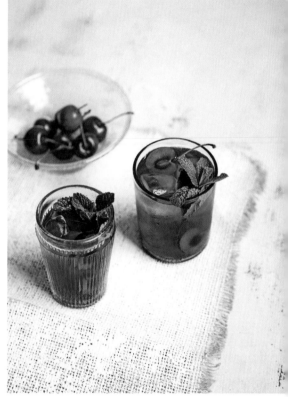

POMEGRANATE & GINGER

INGREDIENTS
1 pomegranate
2 thumbs of ginger
5 cups of water
ice, optional

METHOD
Lightly roll the pomegranate over a hard surface with your hand to loosen the seeds. Slice the pomegranate in half, hold one half over a bowl with the cut side facing down, then bash the skin with a rolling pin or wooden spoon to release the seeds. You'll then have to tear the pomegranate half to pick out the few remaining seeds. Repeat with the other half.

Lightly crush the pomegranate seeds in a pestle and mortar, then scrape them into a large jug along with their juice. Thinly slice the ginger, add this to the pomegranate, then pour in the cold water. Leave to infuse in the fridge for at least two hours before drinking.

TIP
When buying pomegranates, look for those with unblemished, smooth skins and handle them to check their weight – the heavier they are, the juicier they will be.

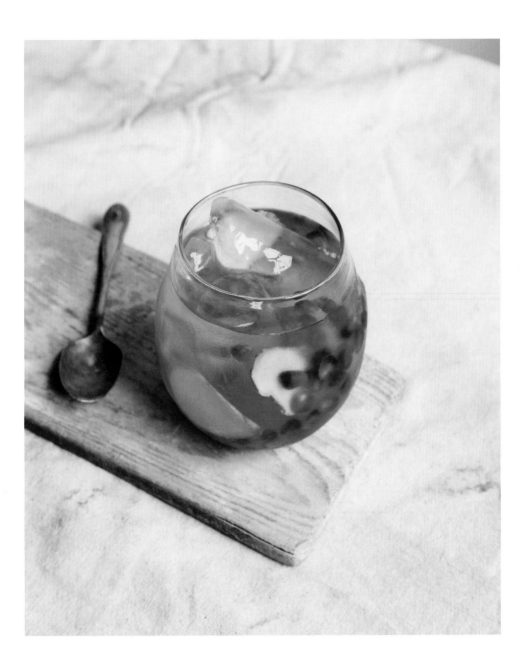

PINK GRAPEFRUIT & ROSEMARY

INGREDIENTS
1 pink grapefruit
6 sprigs of rosemary,
    plus extra for serving
    if desired
5 cups of water
ice, optional

METHOD
Finely zest the grapefruit and sprinkle this into a large jug along with the sprigs of rosemary. Cut the grapefruit into wedges and add it to the jug. Fill the jug with the cold water and leave to infuse in the fridge for at least two hours. Serve with a sprig of rosemary in each glass, if you like.

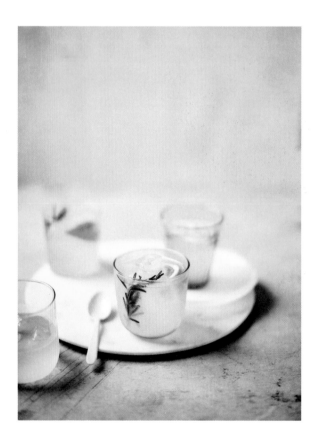

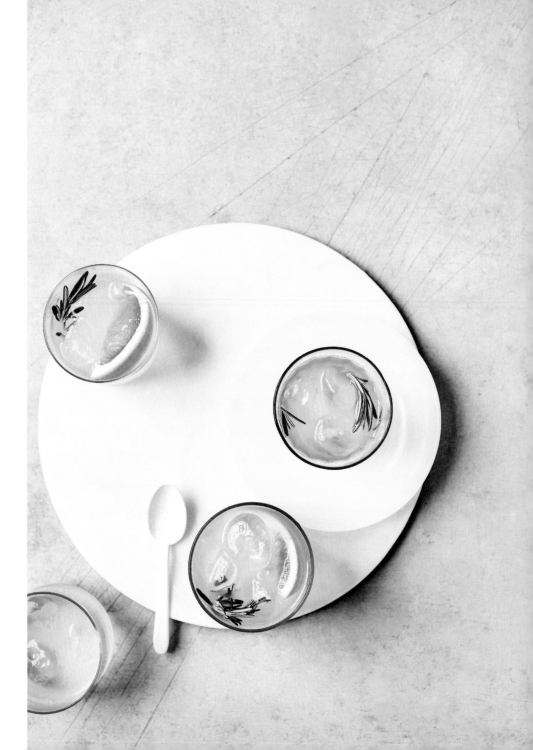

BEETROOT, LEMON & MINT

INGREDIENTS
1 raw beetroot (beet)
1 lemon
3 sprigs of mint, plus
    extra for serving
    if desired
5 cups of water

METHOD
Thinly slice the beetroot and place it in a large jug. Slice the lemon and add it to the beetroot. Lightly crush the sprigs of mint in your hands to release their fragrance, then pop them in the jug. Add the cold water and leave to infuse in the fridge for at least two hours. When serving, garnish with a sprig of mint, if you like.

TIP
Try using up any leftover beetroot (beets) by quick pickling them. Heat 4 tbsp of white wine vinegar with 2 tbsp caster (superfine) sugar and a pinch of salt in a small saucepan over a low heat until the sugar has dissolved. Peel one medium beetroot and cut it into matchsticks, mix it through the sugar, salt and vinegar mixture and leave to cool before serving. Great in salads or as part of a ploughman's lunch.

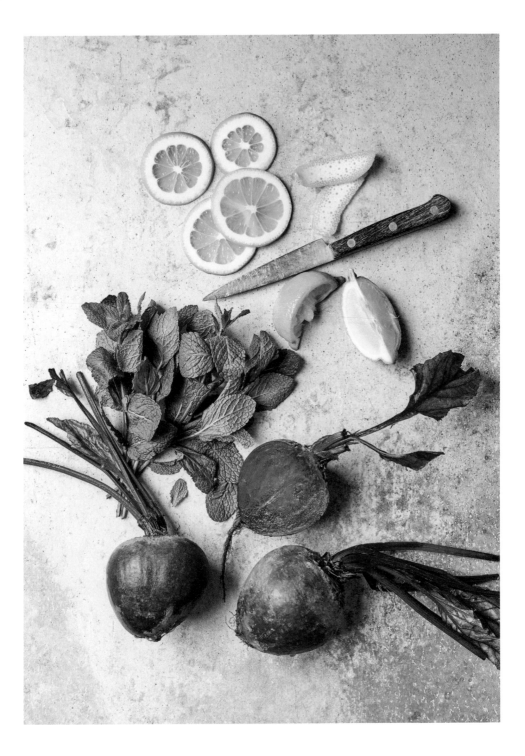

STRAWBERRY, MINT & CUCUMBER

INGREDIENTS
10 strawberries
$\frac{1}{2}$ a cucumber
6 sprigs of mint
5 cups of water

METHOD
Hull and halve the strawberries and place them in a large jug. Using a peeler, slice the cucumber lengthways into ribbons and scatter them into the jug along with the strawberries. Lightly crush the sprigs of mint in your hands to release their fragrance then add them to the jug, too. Fill the jug with the cold water and leave to infuse in the fridge for at least two hours before drinking.

TIP
Experiment with using dried peppermint if you can't get hold of fresh mint leaves.

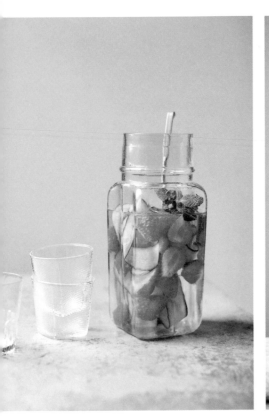

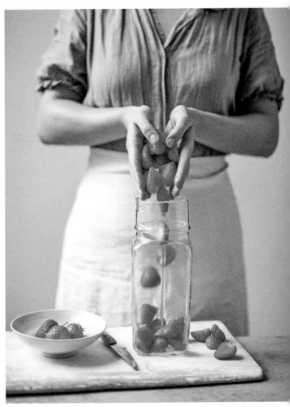

PASSION FRUIT & LIME

INGREDIENTS
2 passion fruit
1 lime
5 cups of water
ice, optional

METHOD
Slice both passion fruit in half and scoop the flesh and seeds into a large jug. Squeeze the juice of one half of the lime over the passion fruit seeds, then thinly slice the remaining half and add this to the jug. Fill the jug with the cold water and leave to infuse in the fridge for at least two hours before drinking.

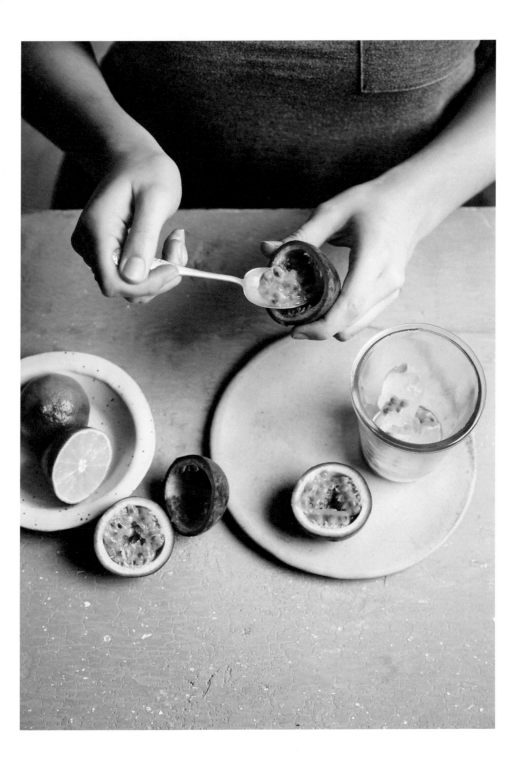

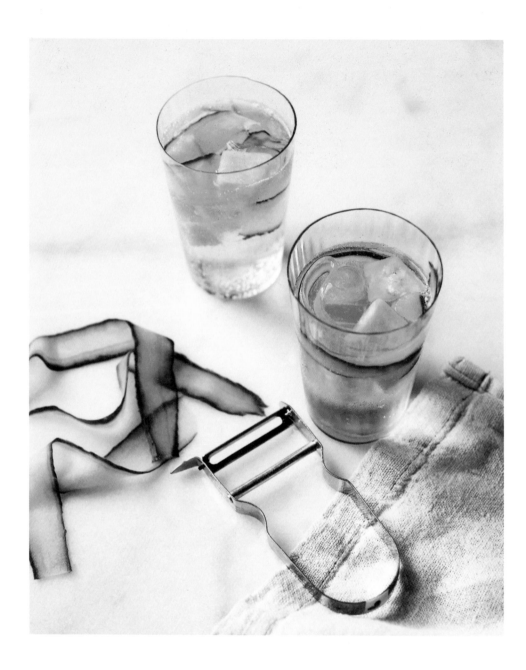

PINEAPPLE & CUCUMBER

INGREDIENTS
$\frac{1}{2}$ a pineapple
$\frac{1}{2}$ a cucumber
5 cups of sparkling water
ice, optional

METHOD
Remove the skin, chop the pineapple into small chunks and place in a large jug. Using a peeler, slice the cucumber lengthways into ribbons and add to the pineapple. Fill the jug with the sparkling water and leave to infuse in the fridge for at least two hours. Serve with a ribbon of cucumber and some pineapple in each glass.

STRAWBERRY, BASIL & LEMON

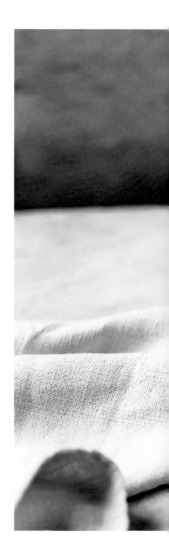

INGREDIENTS
1 lemon
10 strawberries
5 large basil leaves, plus extra for serving if desired
5 cups of water
ice, optional

METHOD
Zest the lemon and sprinkle it into a large jug. Slice the lemon in half, squeeze the juice of one half into the jug and slice the remaining half into thin slices, adding them to the jug, too. Halve the strawberries and add them to the lemon along with the basil. Fill the jug with the cold water and leave to infuse in the fridge for at least two hours. Garnish each glass with a sprig of basil before serving, if you like.

TIP
Try substituting the basil with Thai basil to create an Asian-inspired infusion.

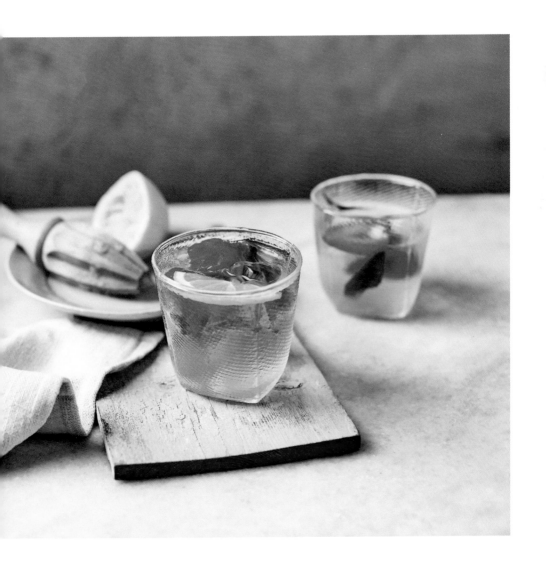

STAR ANISE &
BLACK PEPPER

HOT

INGREDIENTS
1 tbsp black peppercorns
4 star anise
1 tbsp runny honey
2 cups of boiling water

METHOD
Roughly crush the peppercorns using a pestle and mortar, then scatter them in a small teapot. Add the star anise, then fill the teapot with the boiling water. Drizzle in the honey and stir the contents of the teapot. Leave to infuse for five to ten minutes then taste and add more black pepper or honey if needed.

TIP
This peppery infusion is great for helping to fight off colds and sore throats.

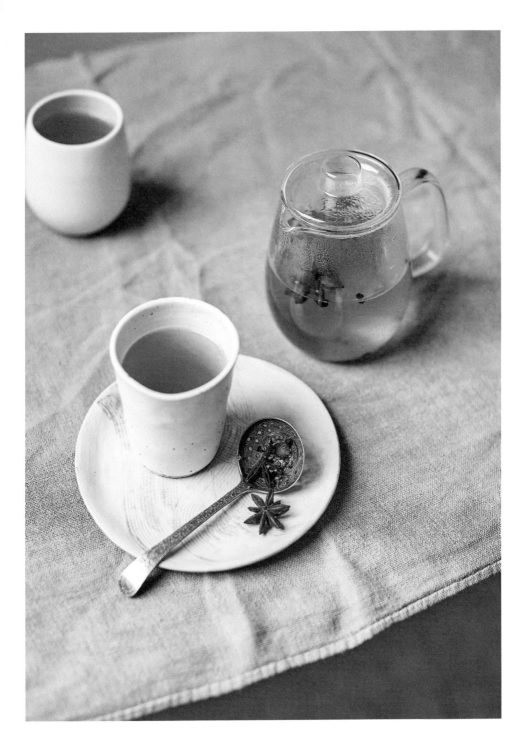

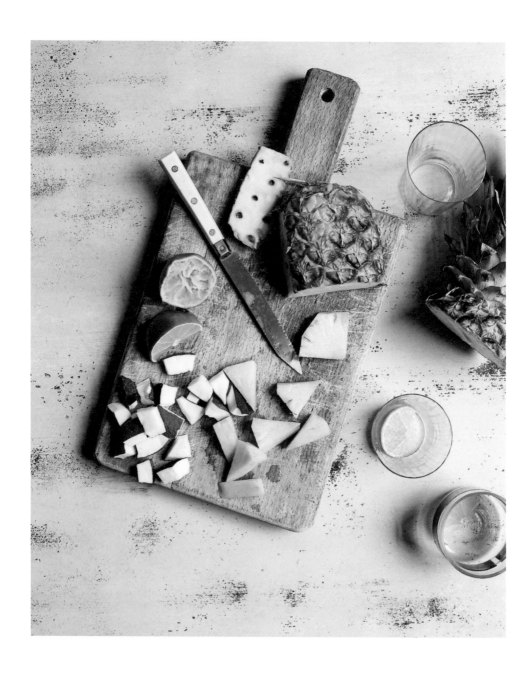

PINEAPPLE & COCONUT

INGREDIENTS
$\frac{1}{2}$ a pineapple
a handful of fresh coconut
　　chunks or desiccated
　　coconut
1 lime
5 cups of water

METHOD
Remove the skin from your pineapple and cut the flesh into small chunks. Place the pineapple and the coconut in a large jug then squeeze in the juice of half a lime. Top up with the cold water and leave to infuse in the fridge for at least two hours. Slice the remaining lime half and pop a wedge into each glass when serving.

POMEGRANATE & KIWI

INGREDIENTS
1 pomegranate
1 kiwi
5 cups of water
ice, optional

METHOD
Lightly roll the pomegranate over a hard surface with your hand to loosen the seeds. Slice the pomegranate in half, hold one half over a bowl with the cut side facing down, then bash the skin with a rolling pin or wooden spoon to release the seeds. You'll then have to tear the pomegranate half to pick out the few remaining seeds. Repeat with the other half.

Lightly crush the pomegranate seeds in a pestle and mortar, then scrape them into a large jug along with their juice. Thinly slice the kiwi and add this to the pomegranate seeds. Fill the jug with the cold water and leave to infuse in the fridge for at least two hours before drinking.

TIP
Pomegranate seeds and kiwis are both excellent sources of dietary fibre, so snacking on the leftover fruits after drinking your infusion is perfect for keeping your gut healthy. Be sure to use the whole pomegranate seeds, rather than just the juice, as this is where all the fibre is held.

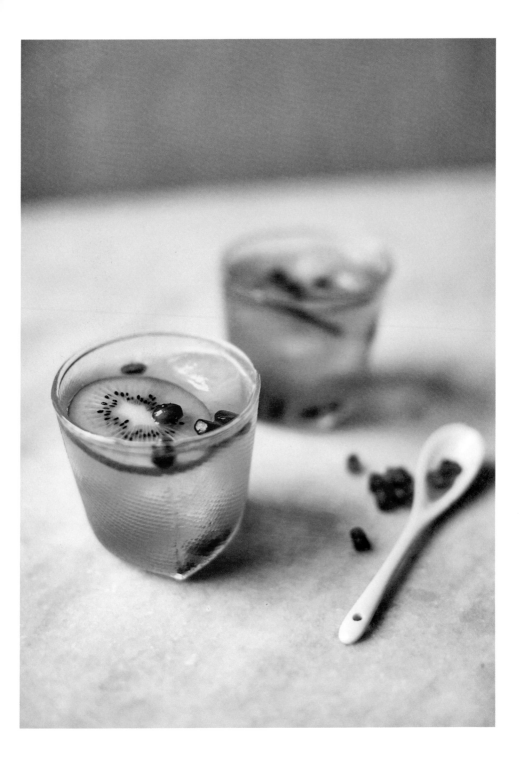

GRAPEFRUIT & RASPBERRY

INGREDIENTS
15 raspberries
1 grapefruit
6 sprigs of coriander (cilantro)
5 cups of water

METHOD
Pop the raspberries into a large jug. Cut the grapefruit
in half, squeeze the juice of one half into the jug and
cut the other half into thick slices – add these to the
jug, too. Sprinkle in the coriander sprigs then fill the jug
with the cold water and leave to infuse in the fridge for
at least two hours before drinking.

TIP
*If you can get hold of one, try replacing the
grapefruit with pomelo, a large and fresh-tasting
citrus fruit from Southeast Asia – similar to
grapefruit but without the bitterness. It has a lot
of pith that needs to be removed with the skin, but
once removed treat it like any other citrus, squeeze
it and use the juice or cut it into slices or segments.*

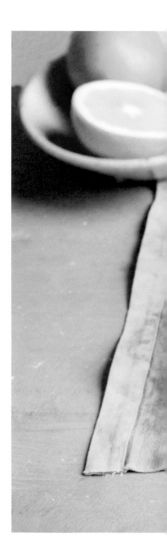

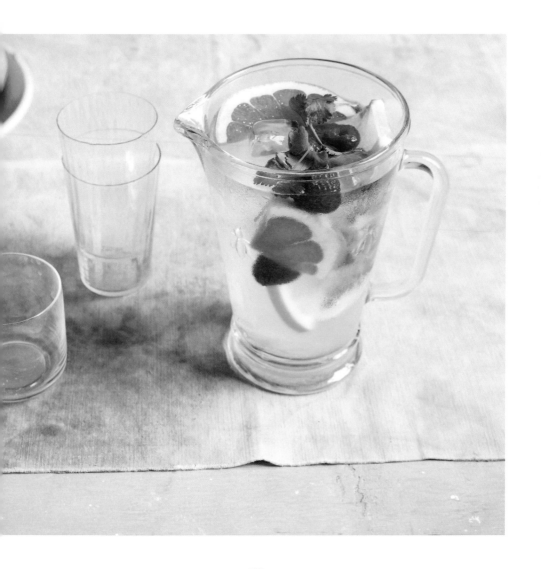

BASIL, PEAR & BLACK PEPPER

INGREDIENTS
1 tbsp black peppercorns,
  plus extra for serving
2 pears
5 sprigs of basil
5 cups of water
ice, optional

METHOD
Roughy crush the peppercorns using a pestle and mortar, then scatter them in a large jug. Leaving the skin on, core then thinly slice the pears and add these to the jug. Pop in the sprigs of basil, then fill the jug with the cold water. Leave to infuse in the fridge for at least two hours. Taste before serving and add an extra sprinkling of peppercorns to each glass, if needed.

TIP
It's well worth crushing whole peppercorns for this infusion as they provide far more flavour than pre-ground pepper.

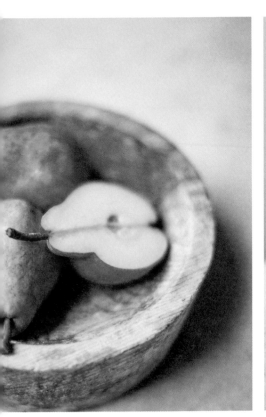
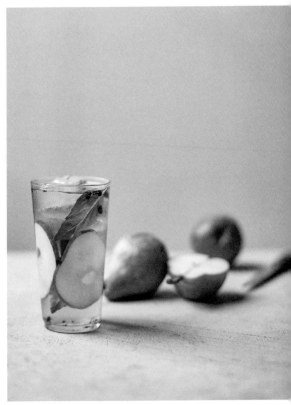

LEMONGRASS & GINGER

HOT

INGREDIENTS
2 sticks of lemongrass
1 thumb of ginger
2 cups of boiling water

METHOD
Bruise the lemongrass stalks in a pestle and mortar to release their natural oils and fragrance, then place them in a small teapot. Thinly slice the ginger and add this to the pot, too. Fill the teapot with the boiling water and leave to infuse for five to ten minutes before drinking.

TIP
Spicy yet fragrant, this is the perfect replacement for your morning cup of tea or coffee.

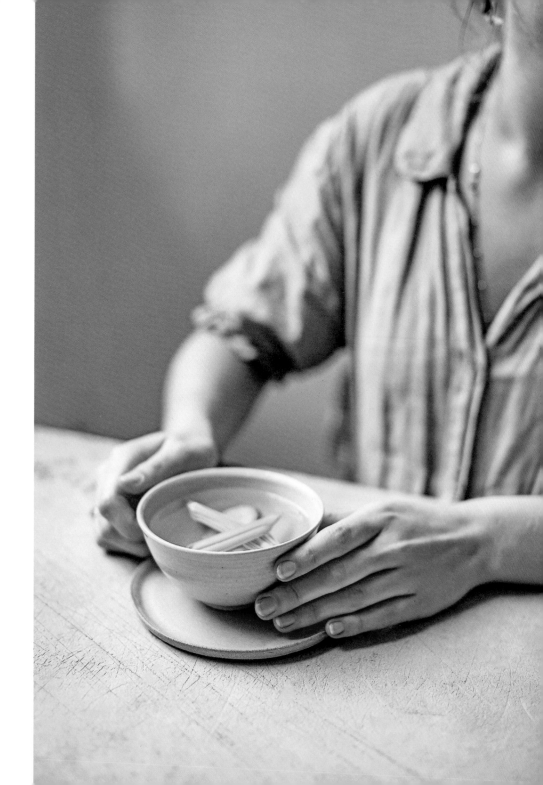

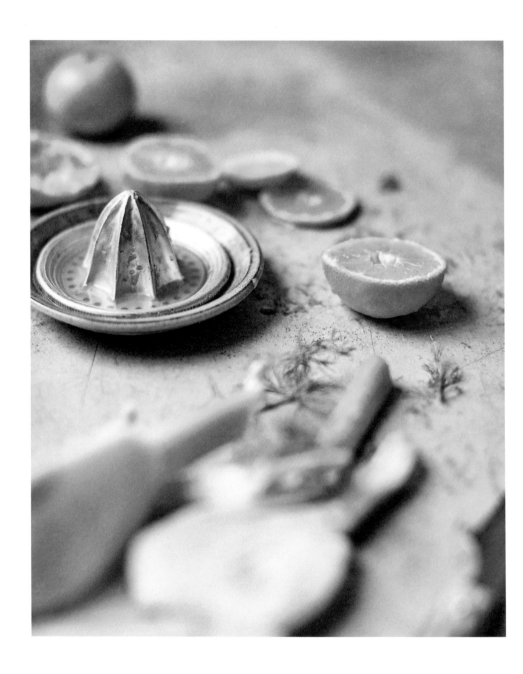

FENNEL & CLEMENTINE

INGREDIENTS
1 fennel bulb
3 clementines
5 cups of water

METHOD
Very thinly slice the fennel bulb and place it in a large jug. Thinly slice two of the clementines to create pretty rounds and add them to the fennel. Juice the final clementine, pour this into the jug, then add the cold water. Leave to infuse in the fridge for at least two hours before drinking. Garnish each glass with a few fennel fronds, if you like.

TIP
Fennel has a variety of health benefits, including aiding digestion and metabolic health. It is also high in vitamin C, so this infusion is a great way to revive yourself if you're feeling a bit sluggish.

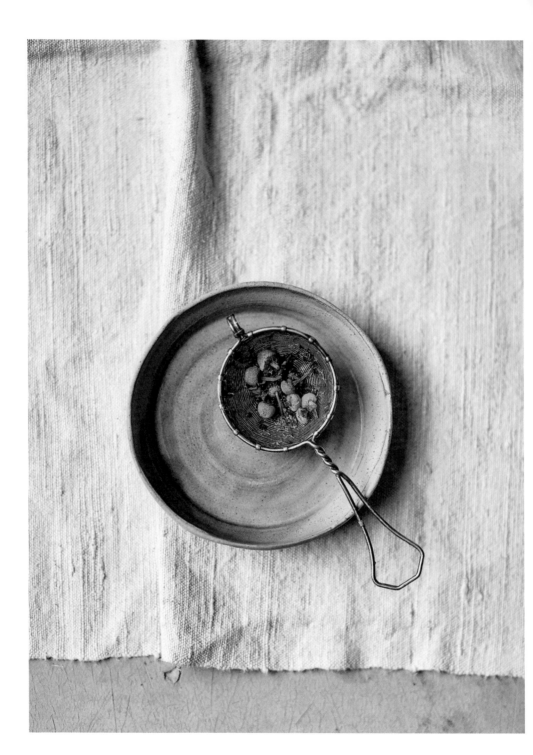

RELAX

Ideal for lazy evenings or weekends, these
recipes use calming, warming ingredients such
as fennel seed and cardamom. Rustle them
up to aid sleep and alleviate the anxieties and
stresses of modern life.

BLACKBERRY & BAY

INGREDIENTS
3 fresh bay leaves
10 blackberries
5 cups of water
ice, optional

METHOD
Bruise the bay leaves slightly in a pestle and mortar, or with the end of a rolling pin, to release their natural oils and fragrance. Cut the blackberries in half and place them in a large jug along with the bay leaves. Add the cold water and leave to infuse in the fridge for at least two hours. Serve each glass garnished with a bay leaf, if you like.

TIP
Bay trees are easy to grow and even do well as house plants, so it's a great idea to welcome one into your plant family.

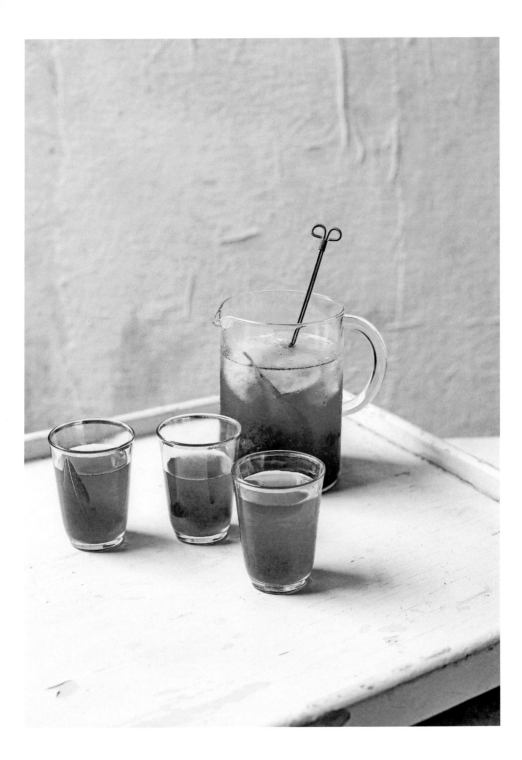

PEACH, MINT
& LIME

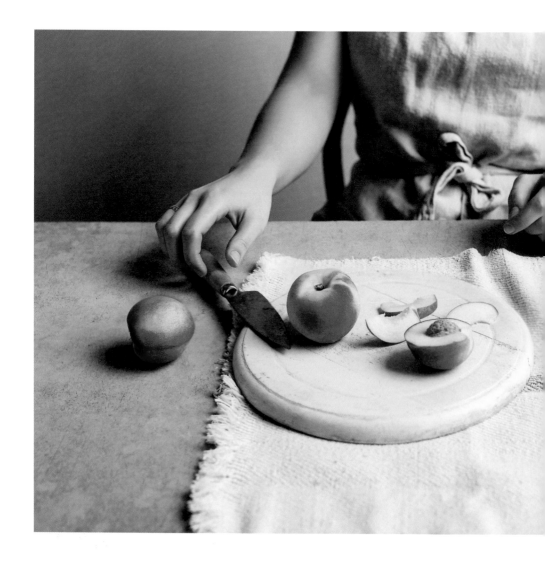

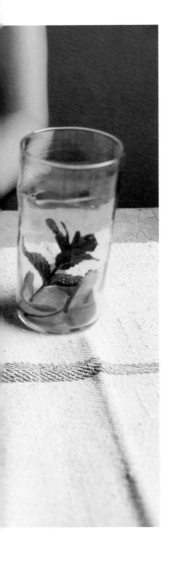

INGREDIENTS
2 peaches
5 sprigs of mint
1 lime
5 cups of water

METHOD
Halve the peaches, remove their stones and then thinly slice them. Lightly crush the sprigs of mint in your hands to release their fragrance, then pop them in the jug along with the peach. Slice the lime and add this, too. Fill the jug with the cold water and leave to infuse in the fridge for at least two hours before drinking.

TIP
Drink this infusion to relax on a sunny summer's day when peaches are at their best. If you can't find peaches, try using nectarines instead.

SPICED RED BERRY

INGREDIENTS
10 raspberries
10 strawberries
2 cinnamon sticks
3 star anise
5 cups of water
ice, optional

METHOD
Halve the raspberries and strawberries and place them in a large jug. Using a pestle and mortar, lightly bash the cinnamon sticks to release their fragrance, then pop them in the jug along with the star anise. Add the cold water and leave to infuse in the fridge for at least two hours before drinking.

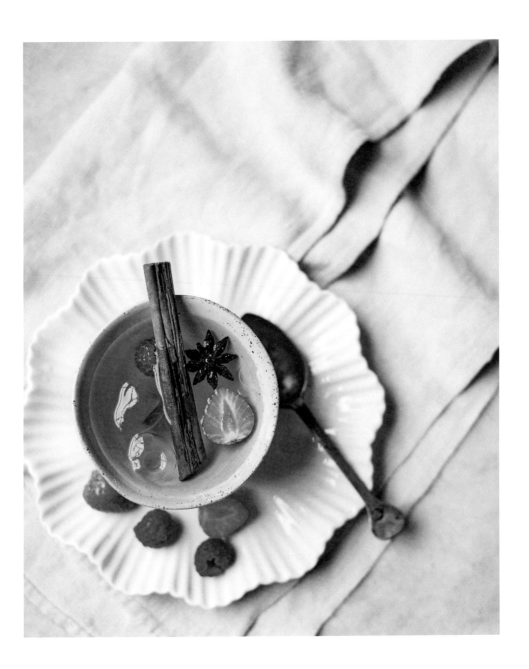

RASPBERRY, GINGER & CARDAMOM

INGREDIENTS
1 thumb of ginger
4 cardamom pods
10 raspberries
5 cups of water
ice, optional

METHOD
Thinly slice the ginger. In a pestle and mortar, bruise the ginger slices and cardamom pods to release their fragrance then tip them into a large jug. Halve the raspberries and add them to the spices, then fill the jug with the cold water. Leave to infuse in the fridge for at least two hours before drinking.

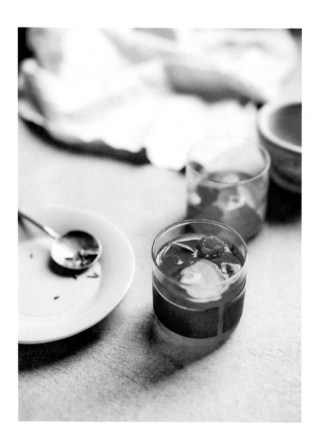

TIP
Cardamom belongs to the same botanical family as ginger and turmeric and so shares the same health benefits of easing digestion and treating nausea. Be sure to freshly crush whole cardamom pods for your infusions; once crushed, cardamom quickly loses its powerful aroma.

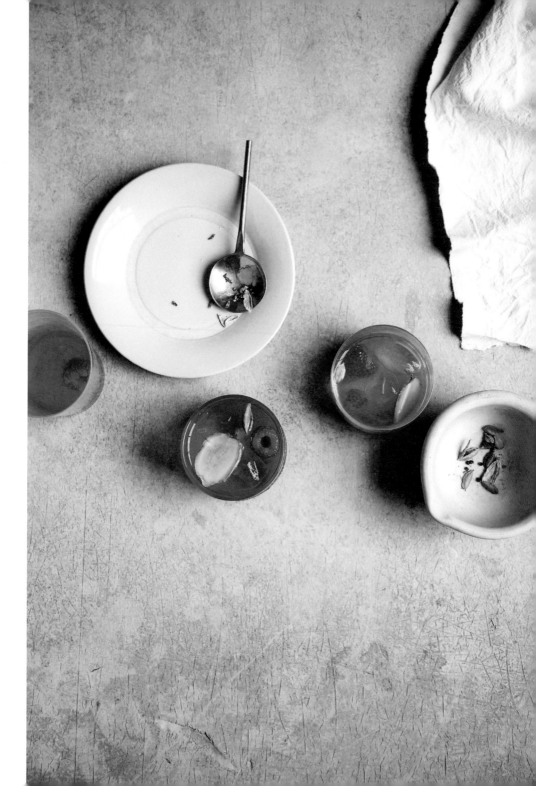

PEAR
& ROSE

INGREDIENTS
2 pears
1 lemon
5 cups of water
1 tbsp rose water
ice, optional

METHOD
Leaving the skin on, thinly slice the pear and place it in a large jug. Cut strips of rind from the lemon using a paring knife, then scatter on top of the pear. Add the cold water, then swirl in the rose water. Taste and add more rose water if you like, then leave to infuse in the fridge for at least two hours before serving.

TIP
For a really special drink, garnish this infusion with pale pink rose petals. Some supermarkets sell edible rose petals, otherwise you can find them in health food stores or online.

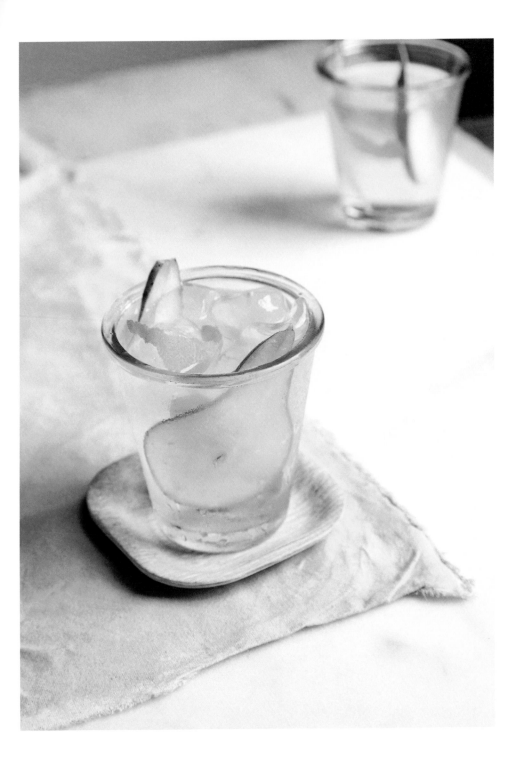

LEMON, GINGER & TURMERIC

HOT

INGREDIENTS
1 thumb of ginger
2 thumbs of fresh
  turmeric
1 lemon
2 cups of boiling water

METHOD
Thinly slice the ginger and turmeric then bruise them slightly using a pestle and mortar to release their fragrance. Place them all in a small teapot. Cut the lemon in half, squeeze all the juice into the teapot, then cover everything with the boiling water. Leave to infuse for five minutes before drinking.

TIP
Drink this infusion first thing in the morning to cleanse your digestive system and kick-start your metabolism.

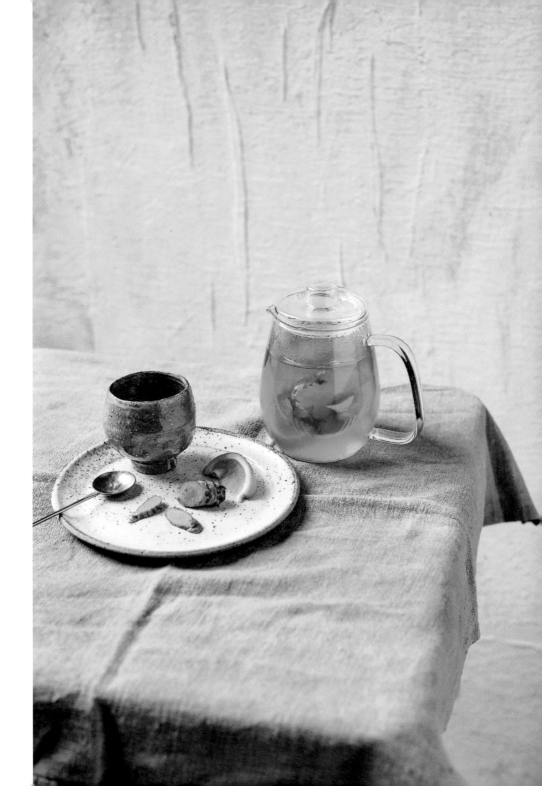

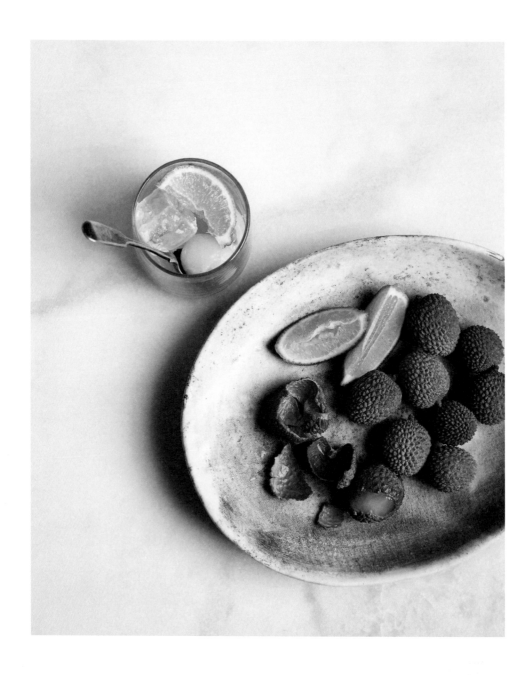

LYCHEE & LIME

INGREDIENTS
10 lychees
2 limes
5 cups of water
ice, optional

METHOD
Peel away the hard outer shell of the lychees, then halve them, remove the stones and place the juicy flesh in a large jug. Slice the limes and add them to the jug. Fill the jug with the cold water and leave to infuse in the fridge for at least two hours before drinking.

TIP
Lychees are high in nutrients like vitamin C, so are the perfect addition to your infusions. The flesh also has a very high water content and is low in calories, making lychees an ideal snack to keep you hydrated throughout the day.

ROSEHIP TEA

HOT

INGREDIENTS
1 tbsp dried rosehips
2 cups of boiling water

METHOD
Put the dried rosehips in a small teapot, then add the boiling water. Leave to infuse for five minutes before drinking.

Note: You can buy dried rosehips online or in health food stores. If you're lucky enough to have an abundant rose bush in your garden, harvest the hips, wash them well, cut each one in half and heat in the oven at 100°C until completely dry.

TIP
Rosehip tea is high in antioxidants, which means it's great for reducing stress and keeping you in good health.

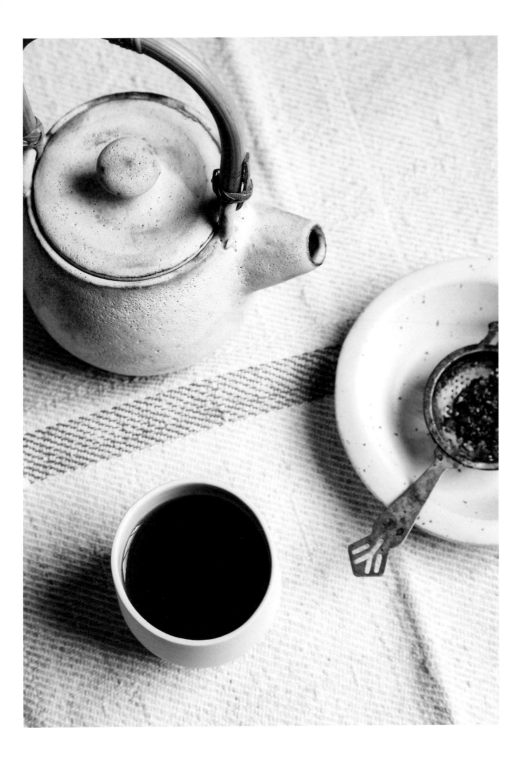

CARDAMOM & ORANGE

HOT

INGREDIENTS
6 cardamom pods
1 orange
2 cups of boiling water

METHOD
Lightly bash the cardamom pods in a pestle and mortar to release their fragrance and place in a small teapot. Cut the orange in half and squeeze the juice of one half into the pot. Slice the other orange half and add the slices to the pot. Fill the teapot with the boiling water and leave to infuse for five minutes before serving.

TIP
Small, Japanese-style teapots make the perfect vessels for hot infusions. Buy them from specialist tea houses or online.

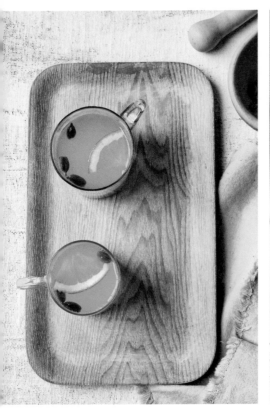

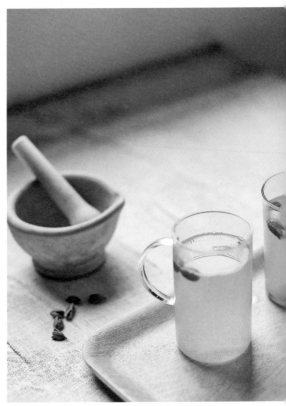

FENNEL SEED & PEPPERMINT

HOT

INGREDIENTS
1 tsp fennel seeds
1 tsp dried peppermint
2 cups of boiling water

METHOD
Lightly crush the fennel seeds using a pestle and mortar to release their fragrance. Sprinkle the fennel seeds and dried peppermint into a small teapot. Add the boiling water and leave to infuse for five minutes before drinking.

TIP
Both fennel seeds and peppermint reduce the symptoms of indigestion, so this infusion is a much better option than coffee for an after-dinner drink.

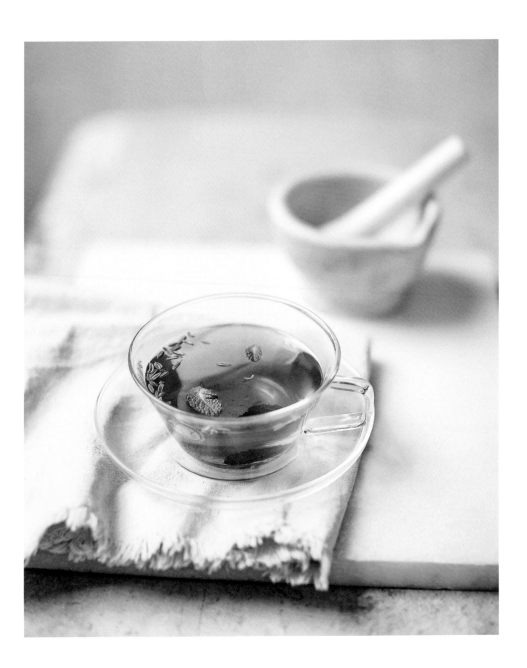

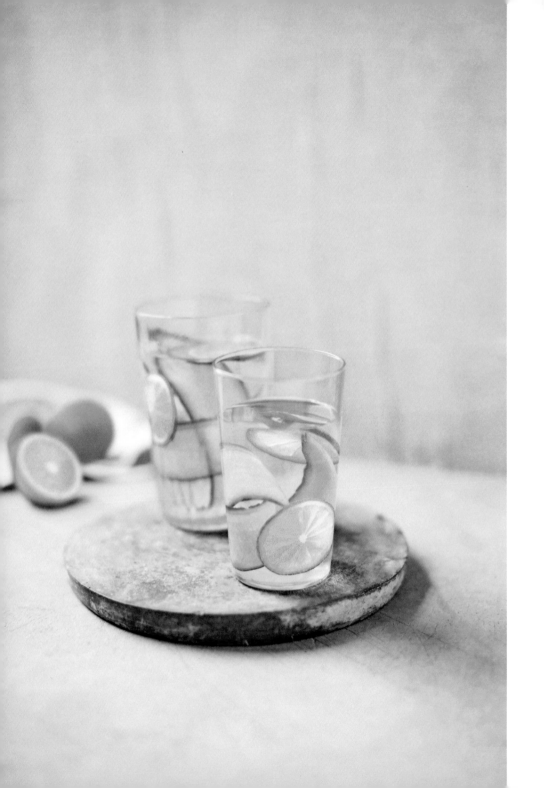

TANGERINE
& CUCUMBER

INGREDIENTS
2 tangerines
$\frac{1}{2}$ a cucumber
5 cups of water

METHOD
Thinly slice the tangerines and place them in a large jug. Using a peeler, slice the cucumber lengthways into ribbons and scatter them on top. Add the cold water and leave to infuse in the fridge for at least two hours before drinking. Serve with a cucumber ribbon and a slice of tangerine in each glass, if you like.

SPICED CHAI

HOT

INGREDIENTS
8 cardamom pods
1 cinnamon stick
4 cloves
2 star anise
2 cups of boiling water
1 tbsp runny honey

METHOD
In a pestle and mortar, lightly bash the cardamom pods and cinnamon stick to release their fragrance, then tip them into a small teapot. Sprinkle in the cloves and star anise, then add the boiling water. Swirl in the honey until it's completely dissolved, then leave to infuse for five minutes. Before drinking, taste for sweetness and add more honey, if needed.

TIP
Steeped in legend, chai is one of the world's oldest-known infusions. Historically brewed as a healing concoction, it has remained one of India's most popular drinks to this day.

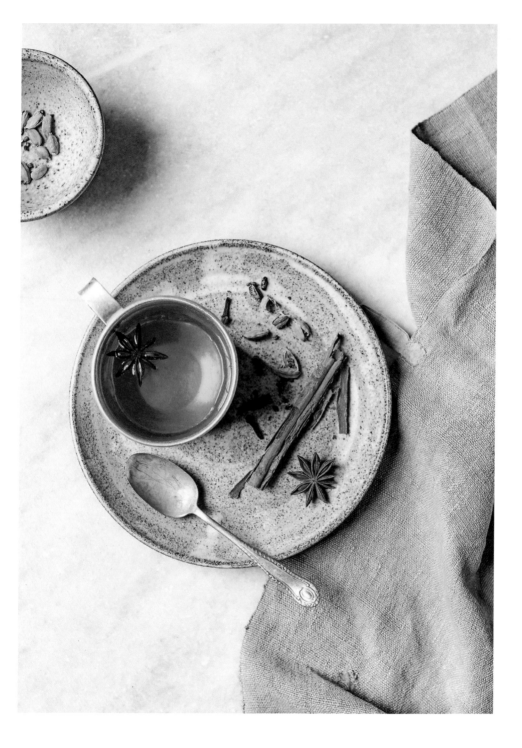

PINEAPPLE
& MINT

INGREDIENTS
¼ a pineapple
5 sprigs of mint
5 cups of water
ice, optional

METHOD
Slice the pineapple into wedges, then pop into a large
jug. Lightly crush the sprigs of mint in your hands to
release their fragrance, then add them to the jug with
the pineapple. Fill the jug with the cold water and leave
to infuse in the fridge for at least two hours before
serving over ice, if you like.

TIP
*Fresh and tropical, this is
the perfect infusion to relax
with on a warm evening.*

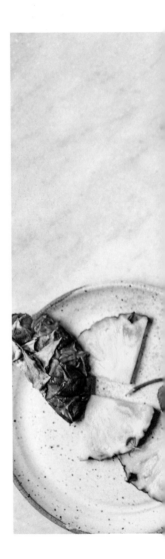

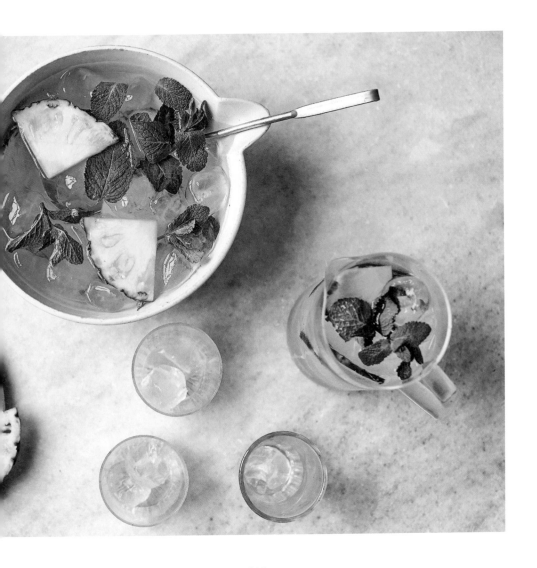

LEMON, BLUEBERRY & LAVENDER

INGREDIENTS
1 lemon
15 blueberries
1 tsp dried lavender
5 cups of water
ice, optional

METHOD
Zest long strips of lemon peel and place them to one side, then thinly slice the lemon and place the rounds into a large jug. Scatter the blueberries over the lemon slices. Sprinkle over the dried lavender, add the cold water then leave to infuse in the fridge for at least two hours. Garnish each glass with a lemon slice, some blueberries and a few strips of lemon zest.

TIP
If you don't have lavender in the garden, you can buy culinary-grade lavender from whole food stores or online.

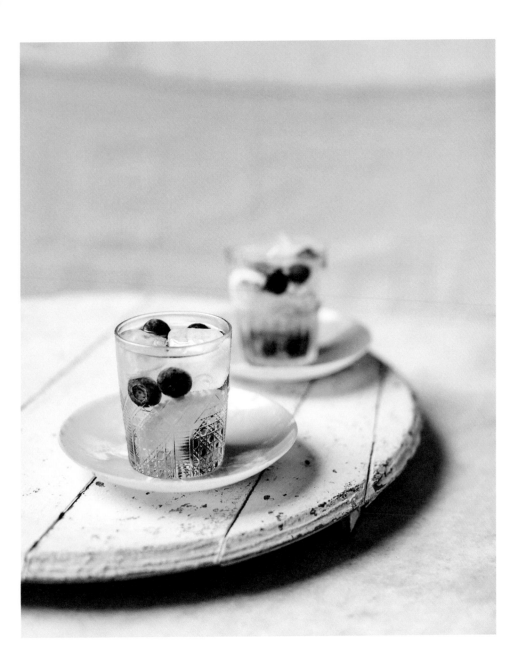

VANILLA, CINNAMON & CLEMENTINE

HOT

INGREDIENTS
1 vanilla pod
1 cinnamon stick
2 clementines
2 cups of boiling water

METHOD
Slice the vanilla pod in half lengthways and scrape out the seeds with the back of a knife or teaspoon. Put the seeds and pod into a small teapot. Lightly bash the cinnamon stick using a pestle and mortar to release its fragrance, then add to the pot. Thinly slice one clementine, then pop it in the teapot. Juice the remaining clementine, add the juice to the pot, then cover everything with the boiling water. Leave to infuse for five minutes before serving.

TIP
Did you know that the vanilla plant is a variety of orchid? Be sure to use fresh vanilla pods for optimum flavour.

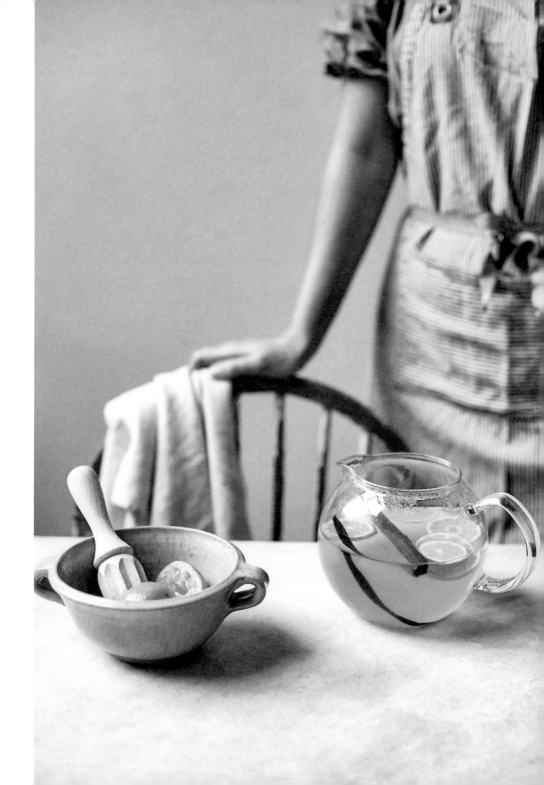

CUCUMBER, LIME & CORIANDER

INGREDIENTS
2 limes
$\frac{1}{2}$ a cucumber
6 sprigs of coriander
  (cilantro), plus extra
  for serving if desired
5 cups of water
ice, optional

METHOD
Thinly slice one lime and place it in a large jug. Juice the remaining lime and add this juice to the jug. Using a peeler, slice the cucumber lengthways into ribbons and add them to the limes. Add the coriander, then the cold water and leave to infuse in the fridge for at least two hours. Serve each glass with a ribbon of cucumber and a sprig of coriander, if you like.

TIP
Fresh coriander is rich in vitamins K and C – keep a pot growing on your windowsill.

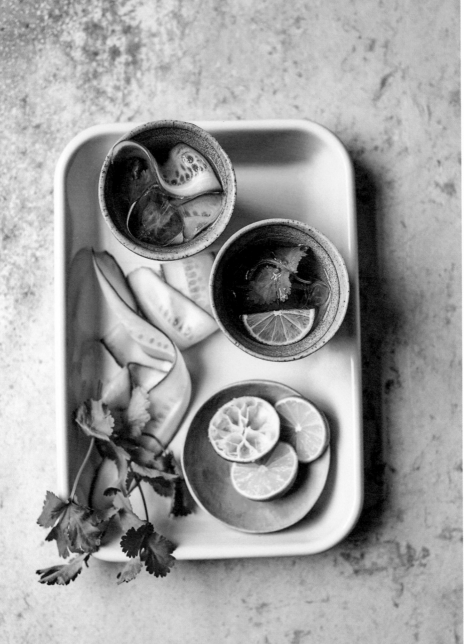

CAMOMILE & LEMON BALM SLEEP AID

HOT

INGREDIENTS
1 tsp dried camomile
  flowers
1 tsp dried lemon balm
2 cups of water

METHOD
Place the camomile flowers and lemon balm into a small saucepan. Add the water and leave to simmer over a low heat for five minutes.

Alternatively, put the camomile and lemon balm in a small teapot, pour over two cups of boiling water and leave to infuse for five minutes.

When ready to drink, pour through a strainer into mugs.

TIP
Camomile and lemon balm promote good sleep, so drink this infusion just before bed for a restful night.

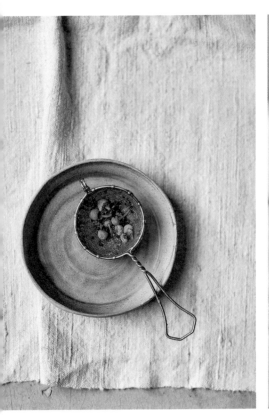

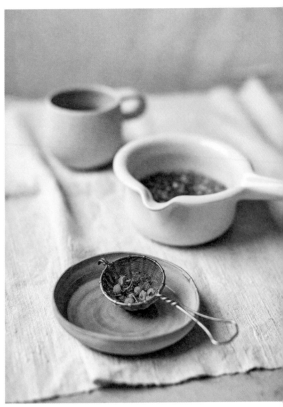

INDEX

HOT INFUSIONS

ACKNOWLEDGEMENTS

Thank you to the marvellous team at Quadrille; to Sarah, Harry and Gemma for firstly asking me to be part of this project but for also always being so easy and fun to work with, ever patient and creative. A special thank you for Harry's special appearance in these pages – I think you'll all agree she makes a great hand model!

To Luke for taking the beautiful photographs that grace the pages and for making this book come to life, and to Louie and her gorgeous prop selection and art direction, for being great company on the shoot and the chats about food, interiors and dogs!

My mother and father for always being the very best support network I could ask for, and for always being at the other end of the phone and, of course, for nurturing my love of cooking from a young age. My sister, Louisa, who is my best friend and eternally kind, positive and helpful and her boyfriend, Pie, who too mirrors that support and positivity always – and thank you for many babysitting hours! My amazing group of girlfriends; Emma, Katie, Kia, Lucy and Zoe, who are, thankfully, eager recipe tasters and always keep me smiling.

Finally (and most importantly) to Tom and my little girl, Louisa, for making this first major project back after maternity leave not only possible but also a real joy to work on. Your support and smiling faces at the end of a long day are invaluable – may cooking for you both continue to be one of my greatest pleasures.

Publishing Director Sarah Lavelle
Editor Harriet Webster
Copy Editor Nick Funnell
Design & Art Direction Gemma Hayden
Photographer Luke Albert
Food Stylist & Recipe Writer Georgina Davies
Prop Stylist Louie Waller
Production Director Vincent Smith
Production Controller Nikolaus Ginelli

Published in 2019 by Quadrille,
an imprint of Hardie Grant Publishing

Quadrille
52–54 Southwark Street
London SE1 1UN
quadrille.com

Compilation, design, layout and text
© 2019 Quadrille
Photography © 2019 Luke Albert

Cataloguing in Publication Data: a catalogue
record for this book is available from the
British Library.

ISBN 978 1 78713 420 1

Printed in China

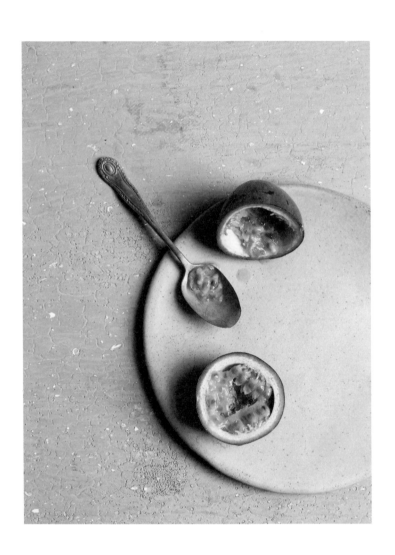